THE Contributions OF Islamic Civilization TO Medicine

The Past and the Present

Volume I

FOREWORD BY

Professor John L. Esposito PhD

Distinguished University Professor of Religion & International Affairs

Professor of Islamic Studies, Georgetown University, Washington D.C.

EDITOR

Mahmood A. Hai MD FICS

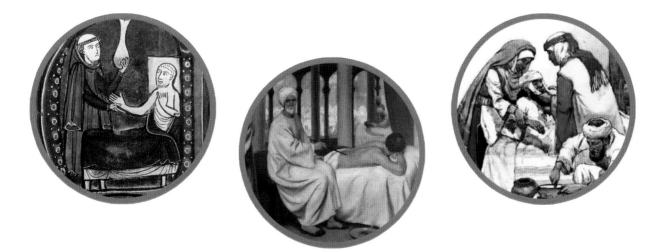

THE ISLAMIC INSTITUTE OF MEDICINE ART AND CULTURE

The Contributions of Islamic Civilization to Medicine:
The Past and the Present

hard cover ISBN: 979-8-35093-255-3
paperback ISBN: 979-8-35092-425-1

Contents

---

1. *Peace Be Upon Him.*

Dedication

Dedicated to God Almighty, the Creator and Sustainer of the universe, the source of all knowledge and wisdom and the Prophet Mohammad (PBUH) who laid the foundation of Islamic medicine.

This book was compiled and published to honor the memory of Dr. Husain Fakhruddin Nagamia, who over many decades laid its foundations before he passed away in June 2021. He spent many years of his life researching the contributions of Islamic civilization to medicine. On his quest Dr. Nagamia visited many countries, libraries, and museums around the globe, till he himself became an authority on this subject. May this book be a fulfillment of his aspirations.

List of Contributors

Professor John L. Esposito, PhD, Distinguished University Professor of Religion and International Affairs and Professor of Islamic Studies, Georgetown University; Founding Director, Prince Alwaleed Bin Talal Center for Muslim-Christian Understanding; and Director of the Bridge Initiative

Mahmood A. Hai, MD, FICS, Retired Senior Urologist, Michigan Healthcare Professionals; Founder and Executive Director, The Surgical Institute of Michigan (Retired); Past Chief of Surgery, Annapolis Hospital, Wayne, Michigan

Tajuddin Ahmed, MD, FACC, Retired Associate Clinical Professor of Cardiology at Wright State University School of Medicine, Dayton, Ohio; Past Chief of Cardiology at The Community Hospital in Ohio

Husain F. Nagamia, MD, FRCS, Former Clinical Professor of Surgery, University of South Florida; Past Chief of Cardiothoracic and Vascular Surgery at Tampa General Hospital, Tampa, Florida; Founder of the International Institute of Islamic Medicine (IIIM) which became the Nagamia Institute of Islamic Medicine (NIIMS) and now the Islamic Institute of Medicine, Art, and Culture (IIMAC)

Ramzi Mohammad, MSc, PhD, Professor and Director of GI Cancer Research, School of Medicine, Wayne State University, Detroit, Michigan

Hossam E. Fadel, MD, PhD, FACOG, Clinical Professor, Obstetrics and Gynecology, Maternal Fetal Medicine Section, (Retired), The Medical College of Georgia, Augusta, Georgia; Past Editor-in-Chief of the Journal of the Islamic Medical Association (JIMA)

M. Basheer Ahmed, MD, FRCPsy, FRCP, Former Professor of Psychiatry, University of Texas, Southwestern Medical School, Dallas, Texas; President, Institute of Medieval and Post Medieval Studies, North Texas

Marium Husain, MD, MPH, Clinical Assistant Professor of Medical Oncology, The Ohio State University James Comprehensive Cancer Center; President of The Islamic Medical Association of North America (IMANA)

Sharif Kaf al-Ghazal, MD, MCh.RCS (Plast.), DM, MA, Consultant Plastic, Reconstructive and Hand surgeon; Plastic Surgery Lead at Bradford Teaching Hospitals in West Yorkshire, UK.
Editor-in-Chief of the Journal of the British Islamic Medical Association (JBIMA)

Fatima M. Tourk, BS, Mechanical Engineering student at Northeastern University

Mubin I. Syed, MD, FSIR, FACR, Clinical Associate Professor of Radiological Sciences, Boonshoft School of Medicine, Wright State University, Dayton, Ohio; Former President, Dayton Interventional Radiology

Feras Deek, MS, Consultant in Physiology and Neuroscience

Azim Shaikh, MD, MBA, CEO, Riverview Health Institute, Dayton, Ohio

Acknowledgments

This book took several years to come together, due to multiple factors beyond our control.

The primary vision came from Dr. Husain Nagamia who was instrumental in doing the initial research, approaching all the contributing authors, and setting the guidelines for this project.

My debt to Professor John Esposito can never be repaid, for he took this work under his wing and lit the path through the dark woods of history. All the contributing editors, who are friends and professional colleagues, form the foundation of this book. We owe our gratitude to the scholars who took time from their busy schedules to review the book with a special mention of Michael Wolfe's untiring effort of an extensive corrective editing. I am especially grateful to Dr. Mubin Syed for contributing a most important chapter on 'Modern Muslim Heroes of Medicine' and holding my hand through the entire editing and publishing process. Great encouragement and support were provided by the Board of the Islamic Institute of Medicine, Art, and Culture (IIMAC), the organization responsible for this publication. Dr. Tajuddin Ahmed and Dr. Shahab Uddin need special mention. I am grateful to my son, Yusuf Hai, for guiding me through the technical steps of putting the manuscript together.

May God accept all our efforts by spreading this knowledge.

Mahmood A. Hai, MD, FICS

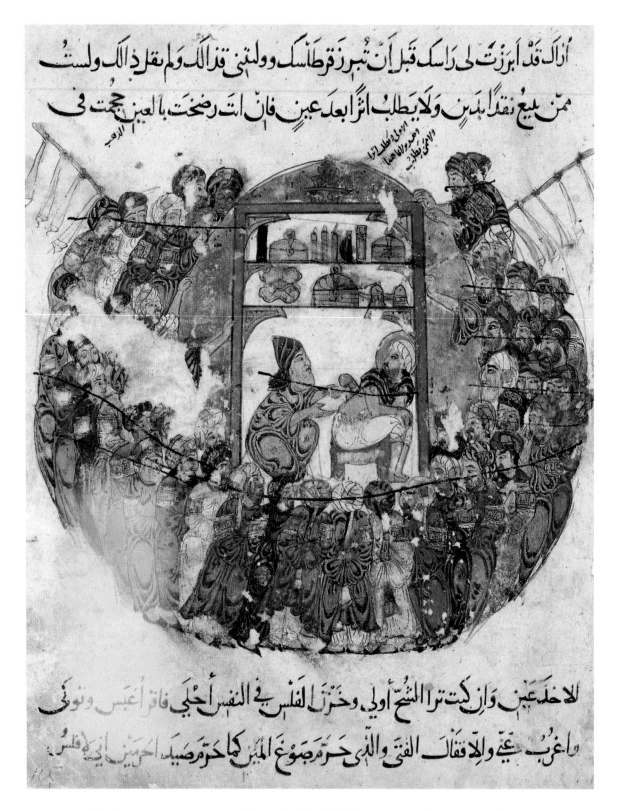

A physician treats wounds in the Twelfth Century: Illustration from
Maqamat, a collection of Islamic tales. (Getty Images).

Foreword

Professor John L. Esposito, PhD

The developmental impact of Islamic civilization on Western science, medical technology, and the arts between the years AD 650 and AD 1450 was enormously significant. Islamic civilization had begun in Medina and was carried on by the Umayyads in Damascus. The Abbasids came to power in 750 under the banner of Islam, legitimating their seizure of authority and dynastic reign.

The early centuries of Abbasid rule were marked by an unparalleled splendor and economic prosperity whose magnificence came to be immortalized in *Arabian Nights* (*One Thousand and One Nights*), with its legendary exploits of the exemplary caliph Harun al-Rashid (reigned 786–809). In a departure from the past, Abbasid success was based not on conquest, but on trade, commerce, industry, and agriculture. The enormous wealth and resources of the Abbasid caliphs enabled them to become great patrons of religion, science, art, and culture and thus to create the more significant and lasting legacy of the Abbasid period, the golden era of Islamic civilization.

The development of Islamic law, Shariah, constituted the Abbasids' greatest contribution to Islam. The Abbasids gave substantial support to legal development. The early law schools, founded during the late Umayyad period (ca. 720), flourished under the caliphal patronage of the *ulama* (religious scholars). By the eighth century the *ulama* had become a professional elite of religious leaders, a distinct social class within Muslim society. Their prestige and authority rested on a reputation for learning in Islamic studies: the Quran, traditions of the Prophet, and law. Because of their expertise, they became the jurists, theologians, and educators of Muslim society, the interpreters and guardians of Islamic law and tradition.

The Abbasids were also committed patrons of culture and the arts. Arabic language and tradition penetrated and modified the cultures of conquered territories. Arabic displaced local languages—Syriac, Aramaic, Coptic, and Greek—becoming the language (lingua franca) of common discourse, government, and culture throughout much of the empire. Arabic was no longer solely the language of Muslims from Arabia but the language of literature and public discourse for the multiethnic group of new Arabic-speaking peoples, especially the large number of non-Arab converts, many of whom were Persian.

Major translation centers were created. From the seventh to the ninth centuries, manuscripts were obtained from the far reaches of the empire and beyond and translated from their original languages (Sanskrit,

Greek, Latin, Syriac, Coptic, and Persian) into Arabic. Thus, the best works of literature, philosophy, and the sciences from other cultures were made accessible: those by Aristotle, Plato, Galen, Hippocrates, Euclid, and Ptolemy. The genesis of Islamic civilization was indeed a collaborative effort, incorporating the learning and wisdom of many cultures and languages.

As in government administration, Christians and Jews, who had been the intellectual and bureaucratic backbone of the Persian and Byzantine Empires, participated in the process along with Muslims. This "ecumenical" effort was evident at Caliph al-Mamun's (reigned 813–833) House of Wisdom and at the translation center headed by renowned scholar Hunayn Ibn Ishaq, a Nestorian Christian. This period of translation and assimilation was followed by one of Muslim intellectual and artistic creativity. It made Arabic the most important scientific language of the world for many centuries and preserved knowledge that might otherwise have been lost forever.

Muslims ceased to be merely disciples and became masters, in the process producing an Islamic civilization dominated by the Arabic language and Islam's view of life: "It was these two things, their language and their faith, which were the great contribution of the Arab invaders to the new and original civilization which developed under their aegis." Major contributions were made in many fields: literature and philosophy, algebra and geometry, science and medicine, art and architecture. Towering intellectual giants dominated this period: al-Razi (865–925), al-Farabi (d. 950), Ibn Sina (known as Avicenna, 980–1037), Ibn Rushd (known as Averroes, d. 1198), al-Biruni (973–1048), and al-Ghazali (d. 1111). Islam had challenged the world politically; it now did so culturally.

Great urban cultural centers in Cordoba, Baghdad, Cairo, Nishapur, and Palermo emerged and eclipsed Christian Europe, which was bogged down in the Dark Ages. The activities of these centers were reflected in the development of philosophy and science.

Islamic philosophy was the product of a successful transplant from Greek to Islamic soil, where it flourished from the ninth to the twelfth centuries. Muslim philosophers appropriated Hellenistic thought (Aristotle, Plato, Plotinus), wrote commentaries, and extended the teachings and insights of Greek philosophy within an Islamic context and worldview. The result was an Islamic philosophy indebted to Hellenism but with its own Islamic character. Its contribution was of equal importance to the West. Islamic philosophy became the primary vehicle for the transmission of Greek philosophy to medieval Europe.

The West would later reappropriate its lost heritage as European scholars traveled to major centers of Islamic learning, retranslating the Greek philosophers and learning from the writings of their great Muslim disciples: men like al-Farabi, known as "the second teacher or master" (the first being Aristotle), Ibn Sina (Avicenna), and Ibn Rush (Averroes), remembered as "the great commentator" on Aristotle. Thus, we find many of the great medieval Christian philosophers and theologians (Albert the Great, Thomas Aquinas, Abelard, Roger Bacon, Duns Scotus) acknowledging their intellectual debt to their Muslim predecessors.

The enormous accomplishments of Islamic philosophy, science, and medicine were the product of men of genius, multitalented intellectuals (polymaths who often mastered the major disciplines of science, medicine, mathematics, astronomy, and philosophy). They were the "Renaissance men" of classical Islam. Avicenna's reflections on his own training typify the backgrounds of many of the great intellectuals of this period:

"I busied myself with the study of the *Fusus al-Hikam* [a treatise by al-Farabi] and other commentaries on physics and mathematics, and the doors of knowledge opened before me. Then I took up medicine. Medicine is not one of the difficult sciences, and in a very short time I undoubtedly excelled in it, so that physicians of merit studied under me. I also attended the sick, and the doors of medical treatments based on experience opened before me to an extent that cannot be described. At the same time, I carried on debates and controversies in jurisprudence. At this point I was sixteen years old.

Then, for a year and a half, I devoted myself to study. I resumed the study of logic and all parts of philosophy. During this time, I never slept the whole night through and did nothing but study all day long. Whenever I was puzzled by a problem … I would go to the mosque, pray, and beg the Creator of All to reveal to me that which was hidden from me and to make easy for me that which was difficult. Then at night I would return home, put a lamp in front of me, and set to work reading and writing … I went on like this until I was firmly grounded in all sciences and mastered them as far as was humanly possible … Thus, I mastered logic, physics, and mathematics.

The Sultan of Bukhara … was stricken by an illness which baffled the physicians … I appeared before him and joined them in treating him and distinguished myself in his service.

One day I asked his permission to go into their library, look at their books, and read the medical ones … I went into a palace of many rooms, each with trunks full of books, back-to-back. In one room there were books on Arabic and poetry, in another books on jurisprudence, and similarly in each room books on a single subject. I … asked for those I needed … read these books, made use of them, and thus knew the rank of every author in his own subject … When I reached the age of eighteen, I had completed the study of all these sciences. At that point my memory was better, whereas today my learning is riper."

Muslim doctors developed new techniques in medicine, anatomy, surgery, and pharmacology. They founded the first hospitals, introduced physician training, and wrote encyclopedias of medical knowledge. They also contributed to the diagnosis, treatment, and prevention of diseases such as smallpox and measles, and Muslim doctors were the first to incorporate surgery, then a separate discipline, into the study of medicine and to develop its practice and techniques.

Islamic science was an integrated and synthetic area of knowledge. It was integrated in that Muslim scientists, who were often philosophers, physicians, or mystics as well, viewed the physical universe from within their Islamic worldview and context as a manifestation of the presence of God, the Creator and source of unity and harmony in nature. Islamic science was also a grand synthesis informed by indigenous and foreign sources (Arab, Persian, Hellenistic, Indian) and transformed by scholars and scientists in urban centers throughout the world of Islam. Thus, it constituted a major component of Islamic civilization and, in the eyes of many Muslims, was a worthy complement to Islam's international political order. As one Muslim intellectual observed:

"Islamic science came into being from a wedding between the spirit that issued from the Quranic revelation and the existing sciences of various civilizations which Islam inherited and which it transmuted through its spiritual power into a new substance, at once different from and continuous with what had existed before it. The international and cosmopolitan nature of Islamic civilization, derived from the universal character of the Islamic revelation and reflected in the geographical spread of the Islamic world, enabled it to create the first science of a truly international nature in human history."

The legacy of Islamic civilization was that of a brilliant, rich culture. Its contributions proved greatly significant for the West, which in subsequent centuries appropriated and incorporated its knowledge and wisdom. Arab Muslim and Christian scholars in Baghdad, Cairo, Cordoba, and elsewhere translated philosophical and scientific works from Greek, Syriac (the language of Eastern Christian scholars), Pahlavi (the scholarly language of pre-Islamic Iran), and Sanskrit into Arabic.

Arab physicians and scholars also laid the basis for medical practice in Europe. Before the Islamic era, medical care was largely provided by priests in sanatoriums and annexes to temples. The main Arabian hospitals were centers of medical education and introduced many of the concepts and structures that we see in modern hospitals, such as separate wards for men and women, personal and institutional hygiene, medical records, and pharmacies.

Ibn Sina (Avicenna) was known in the West as the prince of physicians. His synthesis of Islamic medicine, *Al-Qanun fi'l tibb* (*The Canon of Medicine*), was the final authority on medical matters in Europe for several centuries. Although Ibn Sina made advances in pharmacology and in clinical practice, his greatest contribution was probably in the philosophy of medicine. He created a system of medicine, which today we would call holistic, in which physical and psychological factors, drugs, and diet were combined in treating patients.

This volume, *The Contribution of Islamic Civilization to Medicine: The Past and the Present*, is a publication of the Islamic Institute of Medicine, Art, and Culture (IIMAC). It offers a unique and distinctive study of the past, told by today's Muslim doctors and scientists, about the incredible and extraordinary history of Islamic civilization and its singular advancement and contributions in the fields of medicine. Much of it took place while the West was mired in the Dark Ages, but its knowledge and legacy would influence Western science and medicine as well as philosophy, mathematics, and art well into the eighteenth century.

What is unique about this volume is that the authors of the chapters on the accomplishments and legacy of the past are, as previously noted, modern Muslim scientists and physicians, men and women, who write with knowledge and enthusiasm for an educated general readership. Moreover, readers will come to know and understand the extraordinary accomplishments and legacy of the past as well as in many cases the accomplishments of modern Muslim scientists and physicians. The net result is an appreciation of the history and legacy of Islamic civilization, its faith, followers, scholars, scientists, institutions, and culture, its contributions to and impact on Western civilization.

John L. Esposito, distinguished university professor and professor of Islamic studies,
Georgetown University; founding director, Prince Alwaleed Bin Talal Center for
Muslim-Christian Understanding; and director of the Bridge Initiative

Preface

Mahmood A. Hai, MD, FICS

Islam is the youngest of all world religions and has become the fastest-growing faith among the three major Abrahamic religions: Christianity, Judaism, and Islam. Based on the World Population Review of 2021, there are more than two billion Muslims worldwide—nearly 25 percent of the world's population—making Islam the second-largest religion in the world exceeded only by Christianity. Islam is a monotheistic religion based on the teachings of the Quran and the Sunnah (life of Prophet Muhammad PBUH). It emerged in the Arabian Peninsula in AD 610 and was preached and practiced by Prophet Muhammad (PBUH) and his small band of followers.

Within 150 years the Islamic empire encompassed Arabia, The Middle East, Iran, Afghanistan, Western India, the North African countries bordering the Mediterranean Sea. Islam's golden age began to emerge with Prophet Muhammad (PBUH) himself in the early seventh century. As mentioned in al-Suyuti's book, *Medicine of the Prophet*, "The Prophet not only instructed sick people to take medicine but he himself invited expert physicians for this purpose." The era continued through the caliphate of the Umayyad and Abbasid dynasties and later into the Ottoman Empire for nearly 1,000 years.

This era of Muslim culture has remained unparalleled in splendor and learning and is known as the golden age of Islamic civilization. Because of the Muslim belief that the quest of knowledge is a religious duty, this golden age was a period of enormous intellectual activity in all fields: history, literature, philosophy, astronomy, chemistry, agriculture, mathematics, science, technology, and all aspects of healing and the medical sciences.

This era was also very fortunate to have had unlimited support from its caliphs (the political and religious rulers) and the ruling class. Many great educational institutions were established starting from the seventh century. Outstanding examples of this were the first general hospital, Bimaristan, founded in Baghdad in 805 CE and Bait-ul-Hikmah (House of Wisdom), established in 830 CE under the patronage of Caliph al-Mamun. Scholars, both Muslim and non-Muslim, embarked on an ambitious "Translation Movement," which over a period of two centuries ventured to translate the classical world's scientific and philosophical knowledge as preserved in Greek, Hebrew, and Latin into Arabic and later into Persian, Turkish, Sindhi, and so forth. Over the centuries centers of excellence were established in Baghdad, Cairo, Damascus, Iran, Spain, and India, where aspiring scholars were given the opportunity to acquire knowledge and to experiment in the field of their choice. The number of polymath scholars possessing a significant breadth of knowledge in different fields, both religious and secular, increased exponentially. Notable among them were al-Bitriq, Ibn Ishaq, al-Biruni, al-Jahiz, al-Kindi, Ibn Sina, al-Idrisi, Ibn Bajjah, Ibn Zuhr, Ibn Tufail, Ibn Rushd, al-Suyuti, Ibn Hayyan, al-Tabari, al-Razi, Ibn Firnas, Ibn al-Haytham, Ibn al-Nafis, Ibn Khaldun, al-Baghdadi, al-Zahrawi, al-Ghazali, and many others.

The Islamic empire was the world's first truly intercontinental civilization that yoking together efforts by people of widely diverse origin, including Arabs, Persians, Indians, Chinese, Europeans, and Africans. Its golden age allowed interreligious cooperation, shared scholarship, coexistence, tolerance, and enhancement for the betterment of humanity. There is historical evidence that during this era, women, too, excelled in acquiring knowledge in religious and secular learning, including law, theology, arts, and the medical sciences. The first university, al-Qarawiyyin, was established by a female scholar, Fatima al-Fihri, in 857 CE in Fez, Morocco. Women played a significant role especially in the field of childbirth and gynecologic medicine and on the battlefields as nurses. Yet, because medical historiography was largely a male domain and the society was highly patriarchal, women's voices reach us only faintly from across the centuries.

The contributions of the Islamic golden age to modern civilization are part of the forgotten intellectual history of humanity. Many, including physicians of today, are oblivious to the rich legacy left by our predecessors. If we look closely at history, especially in the field of medicine, after the advances of the Greco-Roman era, Europe fell behind for nearly a 1,000 years. A revival came after the Renaissance in the fourteenth century, and it was all based on the advancement and contributions of the golden age. Many theories and propositions made by Hippocrates and Galen had been challenged over the years and corrected based on extensive work done by the physicians of that era. Many of the books and treatises written and published during the golden age were translated into Latin, French, English, German, and other European languages. They were used as textbooks for the medical schools (e.g., Padua, Italy) and hospital centers (e.g., Hotel-Dieu Hospital in Paris) throughout the continent and became the foundation of modern medicine. Anatomical and physiological concepts, drugs, procedures, and even instruments of our current era are based on these past achievements.

It is interesting to note that the physicians of the golden age divided medical practice into prophylactics and therapeutics, paying greater attention to the prevention of diseases. Diet and regimental discipline played a crucial role in day-to-day life. They believed food has a direct effect on one's well-being. The six important factors affecting health were the surrounding air, food and drink, sleeping and waking, exercise and rest, retention and evacuation, and the mental state. Modern medicine has come full circle, back to these ideas.

This creative and dynamic era started declining after the thirteenth-century Mongol invasion of Baghdad, which brought an end to the Abbasids' rule. With the advent of the new Ottoman Empire, these creative scientific traditions continued for several more centuries until its subsequent stagnation and eventual collapse in the twentieth century. Among the factors responsible for its decline were political mismanagement by the later caliphs, changes in Islamic philosophy, foreign involvement by invading forces and colonial powers, lack of education, and other economic factors. In summary, for more than 1,000 years Islamic civilization's contributions remained advanced and progressive as it stressed the importance of learning, discouraged destruction, developed discipline and respect for authority, and stressed tolerance of other religions. By following the teachings of the Qur'an and Sunnah, these forbearers recognized excellence and hungered intellectually.

This book is being published by the Institute of Islamic Medicine, Art and Culture (IIMAC) in honor of its founder and greatest supporter, Dr. Husain Nagamia. We pray it becomes the fulfillment of his dream for which he gave his sweat and blood for many years. All efforts have been made to confirm the facts mentioned in this book. It consists of essays written by his friends and well-wishers. Several illustrations have been included as visual aids. Because of the extensive nature of the subject, it has been decided to divide the collected, reviewed, and edited material into two volumes. This first volume is in your hands. It is concerned with historical contributions of the golden age of Islamic civilization as well as contemporary contributions of Muslim scholars, researchers, and contributors to the development and achievements of modern medicine and its associated sciences.

Chapter 1 comprises a short biography of Dr. Husain Nagamia, the founder of the IIMAC, by Dr. Tajuddin Ahmed, who was a close associate and supporter of Dr. Nagamia for forty-five years. Dr. Ahmed, a renowned cardiologist, is well known in the community and is a founding member of many organizations, including the Islamic Society of North America (ISNA), the Islamic Medical Association of North America (IMANA), the Islamic Circle of North America (ICNA), and the Miami Valley Islamic Association.

Chapter 2 features a brilliant and comprehensive lecture Dr. Nagamia delivered at the third annual conference of the International Institute of Islamic Medicine (IIIM) in Birmingham, United Kingdom, on June 30, 1998. His talk lays out the very foundation of the history of Islamic medicine and the contributions of Islamic civilization to medicine and science.

The subsequent chapters focus on those who helped build and sustain the golden age along with their short biographies, including Prophet Muhammad's (PBUH) teachings on hygiene, Islamic psychology, and the ethics of medicine. Additionally, a special section has been devoted to the contributions of female physicians and healthcare workers. This first volume concludes with a long (though far from complete) list of contemporary Muslim Physicians, inventors and researchers, who have spurred the development of modern medicine.

Volume II is scheduled for publication in 2024. It will concentrate on the specific contributions made to each specialty of the medical sciences during Islamic civilization. A special section will be devoted to Prophetic medicine (Tibb al-Nabi), its impact on holistic medicine, and its practice in the modern era. The volume will end with a comprehensive bibliography and reference section, *Inshallah* (God-willing).

May Almighty God forgive us as humans for any shortcomings and accept our humble services. May He make this book full of knowledge and guidance for all people and for all generations. Amen.

Mahmood A. Hai, MD, FICS

Introduction

Mahmood A. Hai, MD, FICS

Medicine as we see it today is the result of the cumulative efforts of millions of people over thousands of years—some we know and others we do not. The torch has been handed from one generation to another, passing to those who have accepted the sacred responsibility for growth and progress. However, it never died away, because if it had, it would have been too hard to rekindle it. Between the ancient civilizations, namely the Egyptians, Greeks, Romans, Persians, Indians, and Chinese, and the Renaissance in Europe, came a gap commonly called the Dark Ages, during which this torch was raised, not by the West, but by the Islamic civilization. The term Dark Ages reflects the situation in Europe between the fifth century and the fourteenth. As Dr. Scott Rank described it, "While medieval European medicine was still mired in superstitions and the rigid Catholic teachings of the Church, the advent of Islam in the 7th century CE, gave rise to impressive growth and discoveries in many scientific fields, especially medicine." This era, unjustifiably, has been commonly neglected and passed over, as if no progress had happened. Nonetheless, this was the golden age of Islamic civilization when art and science flourished as brightly as the midday sun. In this publication we are trying to highlight the important events that took place during this time as well as some of the prominent individuals who have contributed to medicine in our current era.

The Spread of Islam

To acquire a fuller understanding of the development of medicine in the Middle Ages, we need a clear picture of the birth and spread of Islam. This new religion was started in 610 CE in a small city on the Arabian Peninsula by a Prophet named Muhammad Bin Abdullah (PBUH). Muhammad (PBUH) first united the illiterate nomadic Arab tribes once torn by revenge, rivalry, and social injustice, developing a strong nation that experienced unprecedented growth. By the time of the Prophet's (PBUH) death in 632 CE, the Islamic empire had spread beyond the Arab lands. Within centuries Islam had overtaken the Persian and Byzantine Empires and parts of the Roman Empire, expanding into Spain, North Africa, the Mediterranean nations, and, later, all the way to India and China, as well as Sicily and other parts of Europe. (See map)

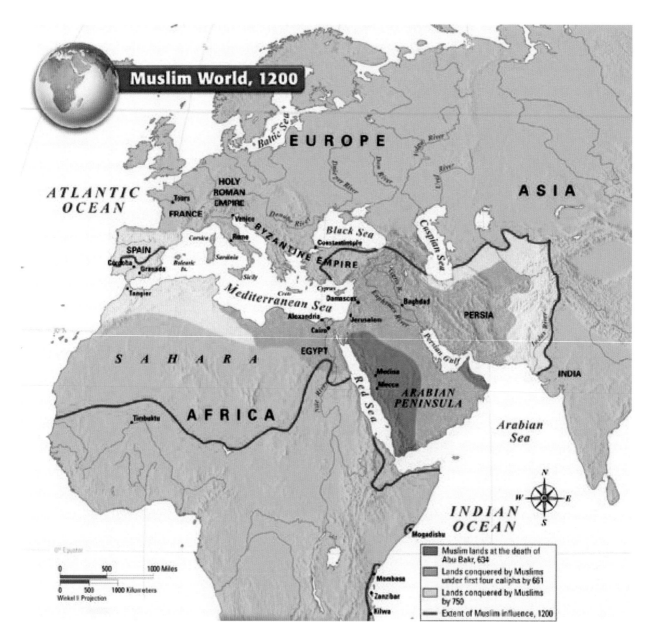

A map showing the Muslim World in 1200 AD

As the new religion grew and expanded it was challenged by the cultures governing institutions it encountered. Unlike other empires, it made determined effort to preserve the cultures and even administrations of the conquered countries. This tolerant ecumenical approach reflected the teachings of Islam, which stressed peace and knowledge, forbade wanton destruction, developed tolerance toward other religions, and promoted authority and discipline. All these factors became the foundation stones of Islamic medicine.

Medicine before Islam

To understand the contributions of Islamic civilization, it is important to evaluate the status of medicine before the change. Classic Greek and Egyptian medicine were not dispensed in designated hospitals; instead, housing for the sick was located adjacent to temples, administered by priests, devoted to divinities said to play a role in the art of healing. In these centers, prayer, sanctuary, and hypnosis were the main forms of therapy. The only highly developed medical school was in Jundishapur (Gondeshapur) in Persia. There, a good part of the medical knowledge was conveyed in the Persian language. In the 6th through the the 9th centuries, physicians associated with this institution like the Bukhitshus, a non-Muslim family, were supportive over six generations in establishing a new medical era.

Features of Hospitals in Islamic Civilization

Contrary to the past, the hospitals of this era were secular in nature and served all people regardless of color, religion, or ethnic background. There were separate wards for men and women, with allocations of wards for different diseases and infections. Male nurses cared for male patients and female nurses cared for females. The hospitals were operated by the ruling caliphate (government) and their directors were physicians assisted by lay personnel. Physicians and staff of all faiths worked together with one aim in mind: the betterment of the patient. To fulfill the Islamic rituals of prayer, clean water was available for ablution and bathing for the patients and employees. Only qualified physicians were allowed by law to practice medicine. There is documentation that in 931CE the Abbasid caliph, al-Mughtadir, ordered the chief court physician, Sinan Ibn Thabit, to screen the 860 physicians then practicing in Baghdad and only those qualified were granted a license to practice. The Baghdadi physician and director of hospitals, Abu-Osman Said Ibn Yaqub, followed a similar procedure in Damascus, Mecca, and Medina. The licensure of legitimate physicians was vital to protecting the Haj and Umrah pilgrims and to curbing the spread of disease among them. For the first time in history, medical care given to patients was documented. The hospitals were not only places for treating patients but also for educating medical students. They were centers for exchanging medical knowledge, performing clinical experimentation, and developing medicine. Attached to these centers were libraries containing recent medical books, auditoriums for meetings, and lecture rooms, as well as housing for students and staff.

During the Islamic era, the science and profession of pharmacy achieved new heights. The vast networks of the Muslim world's global intercommunicating zones, which nurtured trade and travel, also greatly expanded the Arabic pharmacopeia, including many effective drugs and compounds from around the world. Islamic culture's emphasis on seeking the best available treatment when afflicted by disease, and a wide-spread awareness of the core hadiths of the Prophet Muhammad (PBUH) such as "For every disease God has created a cure" supported and encouraged the high standards of hospitals, medical schools, and other health facilities during this era. The general prosperity of the golden age encouraged broad support among generations of caliphs and their elites, who believed that money spent on charity and on building mosques, hospitals and centers of education constituted a good investment that led to immediate societal improvement and granted philanthropists and donors eternal rewards.

Physicians during this era were looked upon with great respect and prestige. Candidates were usually required to complete courses in Islamic studies, philosophy, astronomy, art, and chemistry before being accepted to a medical school. The cream of society's crop, many physicians achieved esteem as polymaths with demonstrated excellence in several fields. They were generally regarded as sources of knowledge and wisdom. In the ninth and tenth centuries the court physician was higher in status than the chief justice. Eminent physicians with the requisite social skills and political capabilities were sometimes elevated to the role of the caliph's prime minister or vizier. Musa Ben Maimun (Maimonides), a twelfth-century Sephardic Jewish rabbi, revered today as one of the chief authorities on Jewish law and ethics, served as personal physician to the great Saladin, the sultan of Egypt and Syria. Because of their high ranks and connections, generous funds for hospitals were easy to obtain.

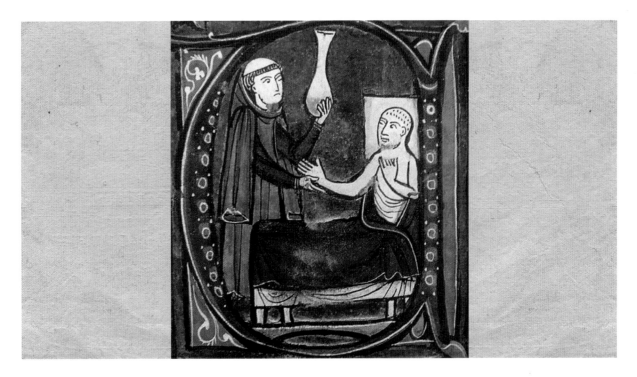

Al-Razi helped establish Bimaristan (hospital) in Baghdad in the late Ninth century CE.

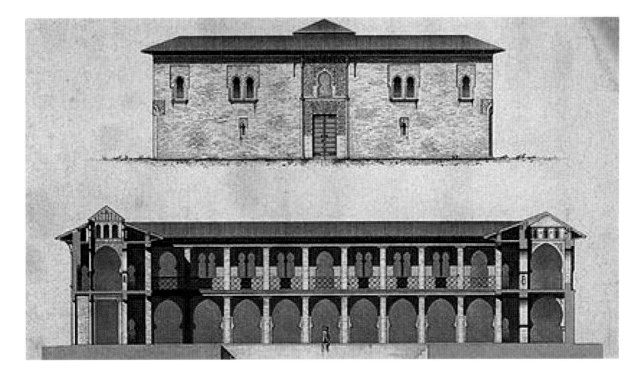

Diagrammatic view of a typical Bimaristan (hospital) during the Islamic civilization.

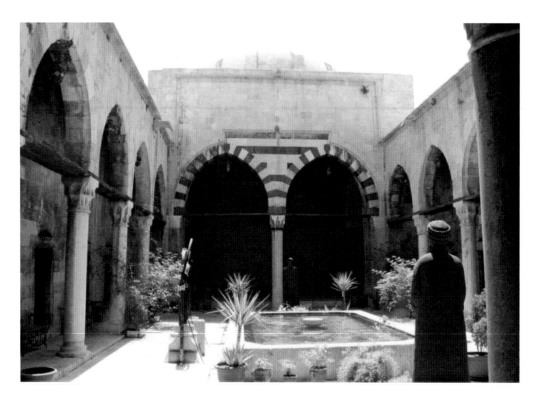

Picture of the interior of a Bimaristan (hospital)

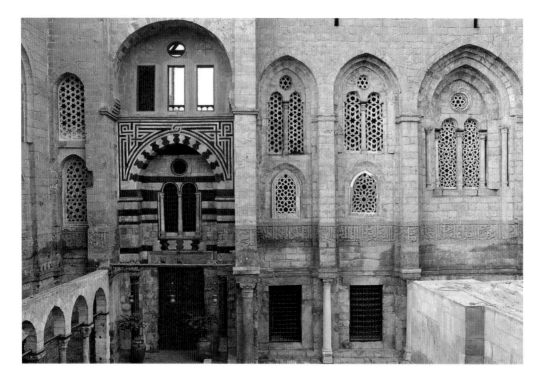

The Al-Mansur Qalawun Hospital Complex in Cairo 1248 AD

Well-Known Hospitals of Islamic Civilization

Since the capital of the Islamic empire kept changing with the ruling dynasty, important medical centers developed in many major cities. The first known hospital of the golden era was built in Damascus in 706 CE by the Umayyad caliph, al-Walid. Later, in 1154 CE, al-Nuri Hospital was built and named after King Nur al-Din Zinki. It became a first-class medical school with a rich medical library and complete patient medical records. Many eminent physicians graduated from this school, including Ibn al-Nafis, who provided the first description of pulmonary circulation. This institution served the people of Damascus for seven centuries. In 1055 CE the Crusaders built Saint John Hospital in Jerusalem. After Saladin's (Salah al-Din) victory in 1187 CE this hospital was expanded and renamed al-Salahani Hospital. It continued to give public medical care until an earthquake destroyed it in 1458 CE. In Iraq and Persia, Baghdad became the capital of the Abbasid dynasty in 750 CE. In 766 CE, Caliph al-Mansur, invited Jurjis Ibn Bukhtishu from Jundishapur to establish a hospital worthy of the prosperous capital. Twenty years later the renowned caliph Harun al-Rashid had a special hospital built under the guidance of Jibril Bukhtishu, the grandson of Jurjis. The hospital was named Baghdad Hospital, and it went on to produce many eminent physicians like al-Razi. In 918 CE Caliph al-Muqtadir added two more hospitals in Baghdad, one on the east side—al-Sayyidah Hospital—and one on the west—al-Muqtadiri Hospital. In 981 CE Caliph Adud al-Dawlah, being determined to outdo his predecessors, built the capital's most magnificent hospital, which was furnished with the best equipment of the day and employed interns, residents, and twenty-four consultants attending to its professional activities. Haly Abbas, the Persian physician and psychologist who wrote a widely used textbook, "The Complete Book of the Medical Art" (*Kitab Al-Malaki* or *Liber Regius*) was on the staff. Unfortunately, the hospital was demolished in 1258 by Holagu, the grandson of Genghis Khan, when the Mongols invaded Baghdad.

In Egypt, al-Fustat Hospital was built in 872 CE to serve the people of Old Cairo. It served the local population for six centuries, before being updated as Mustashfa Qalawun (see picture), an ophthalmology center. (The hospital's ancient doors are preserved in the Islamic Museum of Cairo). Al-Mansuri Hospital was constructed by the order of King al-Mansur Qalawun in 1284 CE. Contemporary traveler and author Ibn Batuta and the historian El-Kalkashandi reported it to be the best hospital ever built. It had separate sections for each disease and served more than 4,000 patients daily. Patients' stays were free and, upon discharge they were given food and money as compensation for lost wages.

In North Africa, known as al-Maghrib al-Arabi, many hospitals were established in different regions. The first, al-Qayrawan Hospital, was built in Tunisia in 830 CE in the city of al-Dimnah. Many other hospitals were subsequently built in other cities in a similar fashion. They were characterized by spacious separate wards, waiting rooms for patients and visitors, and They were characterized by spacious separate wards, waiting rooms for patients and visitors, and a chapel for prayers.

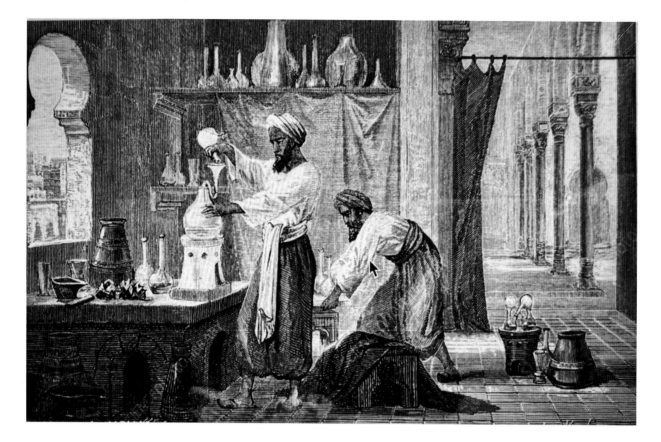

A hospital pharmacy in Spain during the Almohad period

The first hospital in Morocco was opened in 1190 CE in the capital city of Marrakesh by the Almohad caliph Yacoub al-Mansour. Called Dar-al-Faraj, the House of Appeasement, it was a huge facility, beautifully landscaped with fruit trees and fountains providing water supplied by the city's extensive system of aqueducts. The hospital offered an expensive private section for the city's affluent elite, whose fees helped support the rest of its public services.

Across the Mediterranean in Andalucía (Muslim Spain), a training school for physicians was opened in the new capital, Cordoba, in the first years of Abd al-Rahman's founding reign (822-852 CE). There the works of Galen and many other Greek texts were studied in Arabic. By the eleventh century, forty to fifty hospitals flourished in Cordoba, alone.

One of Andalusia's last hospitals were constructed under Prince Muhammad Ibn Yusuf Ibn Nasr in Granada in 1366 CE. It was a beautiful, appointed complex, architecturally, and served the half a million residents of Granada. King Ferdinand and Queen Isabella's Castilian forces destroyed the hospital at the fall of Granada in 1492 CE.

Methods of Treatment Used in the Islamic Era

Classic Islamic medicine provides a holistic approach to health. Among physicians in the medieval and pre-Modern periods, being healthy meant being healthy physically, mentally, and spiritually. Physicians of the Islamic era strongly believed in prevention of diseases, giving great importance to diet, physical activities, and meditation. Treatment started with physiotherapy, which included exercises and water baths. Proper nutrition was an important element too, with an elaborate system of dieting and supplementing food deficiencies. If that failed, the physician would refer the patient to the extensive pharmacopeia that was available. Drugs were divided into two groups: simple and compound. The dosage and adverse effects were experimented at length and documented. If these measures failed, surgery was undertaken as the last resort.

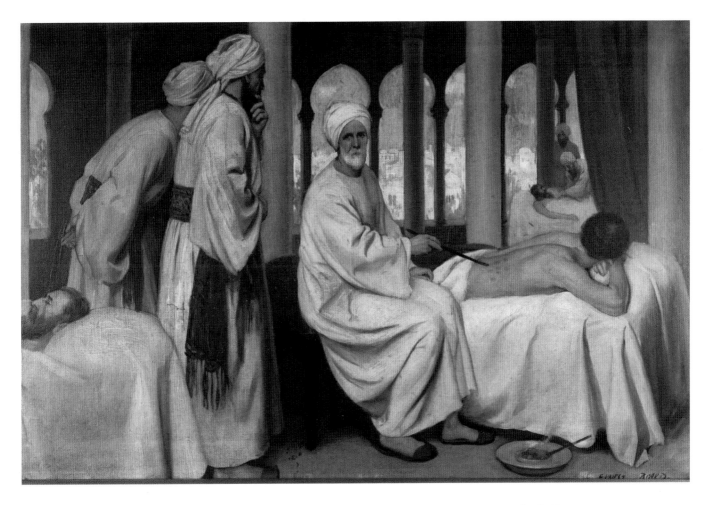

A Muslim physician of the Islamic era treating a patient at bedside.

Medical Ethics Followed during the Islamic Era

Physicians followed a strict code of ethics laid down by their leaders. In 970 CE, al-Tabari, one of the chief physicians of the Abbasid period, described this Islamic code of ethics as follows:

"1. Personal character of the physician:

The physician ought to be modest, virtuous, merciful and unaddicted to liquor (as any form of alcohol was forbidden by Islam). He should wear clean clothes, be dignified, and have well-groomed hair and beard. He should not join the ungodly and the scoffers nor sit at their table. He should select his company to be persons of good reputation. He should be careful of what he says and should not hesitate to ask forgiveness if he has made an error. He should be forgiving and never seek revenge. He should be friendly and be a peacemaker. He should not make jokes or laugh at the improper time or place.

2. His obligations toward patients:

The physician should avoid predicting whether a patient will live or die, only God knows. He ought not to lose his temper when his patient keeps asking questions but should answer gently and compassionately. He should treat alike the rich and the poor, the master, and the servant, the powerful and the powerless, the elite and the illiterate. God will reward him if he helps the needy. The physician should not be late for his rounds or his house call. He should be punctual and reliable. He should not wrangle about his fees. If the patient is very ill or in an emergency, he should be thankful, no matter how much he is paid. He should not give drugs to a pregnant woman for an abortion unless necessary for the mother's health. If the physician prescribes a drug orally, he should make sure the patient understands the name correctly, in case he has asked for the wrong drug and gets worse instead of better. He should be decent toward women and should not divulge the secrets of his patients.

3. His obligations toward the community:

The physician should speak no evil of reputable men of the community or be critical of anyone's religious belief.

4. His obligations toward his colleagues:

The physician should speak well of his acquaintances and colleagues. He should not honor himself by shaming others. If another physician has been called to treat his patient, the family doctor should not criticize his colleague even if the diagnosis and recommendations of the latter differ from his own. However, he has the obligation to explain what each point of view may lead to since his duty is to counsel the patient as best as he can. He must warn the patient that combining different types of therapy may be dangerous because the actions of different drugs may be incompatible and injurious.

5. His obligations toward his assistants:

If the subordinate does something wrong, the physician should not rebuke him in front of others but correct him privately and cordially."

Stages in the Development of Medicine during the Golden Era of Islamic Civilization

Historically there were three stages in the development of Islamic medicine.

I. The first stage involved translation. This began at the beginning of the seventh century and lasted until the end of the ninth century. During this stage Syrian and Persian scholars did a notable job of translating ancient literature from Greek and Syriac into Arabic. The works of Hippocrates (460–370 BC), Aristotle (384–322 BC), and Galen (131–210 CE) were among the important texts translated. Muslim rulers like Caliph al-Mamun encouraged translation and paid the translator the weight of his translation in gold. Among the eminent physicians were Jurjis Ibn Bukhtishu and his grandson Jibril, Yuhanna Ibn Masawaya, al-Bitriq, and Hunayn Ibn Ishaq. Many of the physicians of this period were Christians who received full recognition and renumeration were respectfully given by the Muslim rulers.

II. The second stage was the stage involved with experimentation and subsequent confirmation. This stage extended from the ninth century to the fourteenth. Many prominent physicians, philosophers, polymaths, scientists, and artists of this period contributed not only to medicine but also to every branch of science and art with unlimited cooperation. Those who made the greatest impact and are well documented in history will be discussed in the following chapters.

III. The third stage, from the fourteenth century to the nineteenth, involved the transference of knowledge to Europe with extensive translations of the great classical treatises into Latin, French, German, Italian, English, and other languages. Many of the books became the textbooks of modern medicine and were used until the nineteenth century. At the close of this stage, stagnation and deterioration occurred, finally ending this glorious golden era.

Decline of Islamic Civilization

According to most historians, the decline of Islamic civilization started as early as the later years of the tenth century CE. The decline has been attributed to multiple factors. First, there was a withdrawal of the once unwavering support of the rulers and the affluent of the society. The main person responsible is said to be Abul Hasan Ali Tulsi (1018–1092 CE), better known in history as Nizam al-Mulk. Starting from a lowly position he became a scholar, jurist, and political philosopher and later the vizier of the ruling Seljuk Empire. Many historians view him as one of the most important statesmen in Islamic history and the de facto ruler of the empire for over twenty years. His most important legacy was the founding of the *madrassa* system, the first government-sponsored education system in history. This not only impeded to the progression of the golden era but favored the more orthodox teachings of Islam. Some of the great theologians of the time believed the Islamic spiritual tradition had become moribund, neglecting the spiritual sciences taught by the first generation of Muslims. To protect Islamic philosophy and practice, they and a large group of their supporters reduced the emphasis on the growth of contemporary sciences of that era. By the beginning of the fifteenth century Islamic educational institutions and universities had removed the study of science from their curriculum. Subsequent Muslim empires including the Mughals, the Safavids, and Ottomans could not reverse the decline. The second major setback came with the devastating Mongol attack on Baghdad in February 1258. For the next five centuries Muslim nations were dominated and demoralized by European colonialism.

By the late 1400s European scholars and educators had begun translating Islamic scientific works from Arabic into Western languages like Latin, Spanish, French, and English, installing them as textbooks in their medical schools. In the early twentieth century religious and educational revival and reform efforts were made by Sir Syed Ahmad Khan (1817–1898 CE) in India and Mohammad Abduh (1849–1905 CE) in Egypt, but the glory of the golden era had passed.

Mahmood A. Hai, MD, FICS

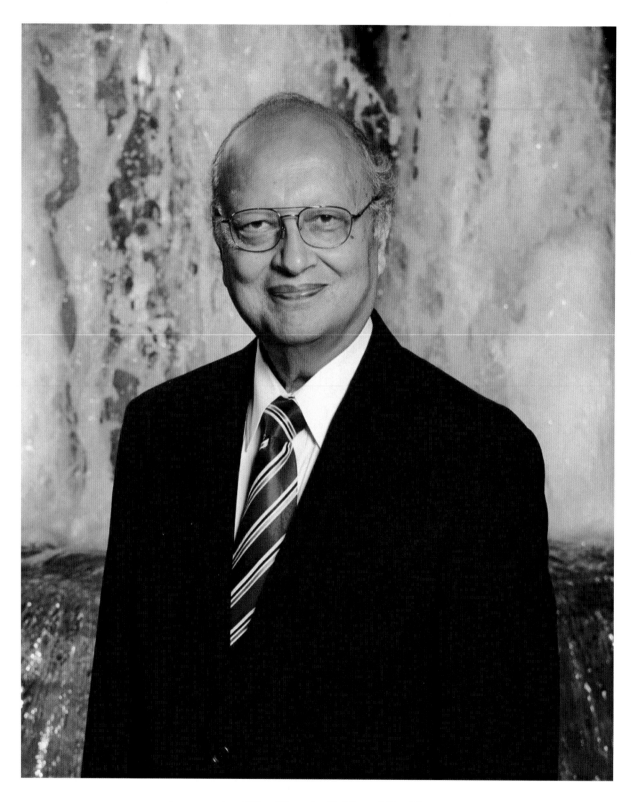

A portrait of Dr. Husain Fakhruddin Nagamia
(Born: June 29,1939 Died: June 4, 2021)

CHAPTER 1:

Biography of Dr. Husain Nagamia

Tajuddin Ahmed, MD, FACC

Dr. Husain Fakhruddin Nagamia was born in Baroda, India, on June 29, 1939, and passed away in Tampa, Florida, on June 4, 2021. He attended St Michael High School in Bombay from 1944 to 1954. He received a scholarship for his medical studies at Grant Medical School in Bombay from 1956 to 1962 and graduated with gold medals and honors. During this era, he had the tutelage of his uncle, who was the principal of Bombay Veterinary College. On October 27, 1962, Dr. Nagamia went to England, where he completed his internship and residency and served as a registrar in surgery from 1966 to June 1970. While in the UK he obtained a fellowship from the Royal College of Surgeons of England and Edinburgh. The same year he accepted the position of chief surgeon at Aramco Hospital in Alkhobar, Saudi Arabia, where he served for two years. Soon after Dr. Nagamia moved with his family to the United States and joined the general surgical residency program at the University of Massachusetts, which he completed in June 1974. He then finished two years of a cardiothoracic and vascular surgical residency at Boston University and served as a research fellow from July to December 1976.

Dr. Nagamia and his family moved to Tampa in 1977, where he established his practice in the Tampa Bay area and practiced diligently for over forty years. During this era, he was on the staff at many neighboring hospitals, including Tampa General Hospital, Brandon Regional Hospital, South Bay Hospital, Memorial Hospital, and Tampa Community Hospital. He served as a clinical professor of surgery at the University of South Florida from 1996 to 2005 and as the chief of cardiothoracic and vascular surgery at Tampa General Hospital from 1998 to 2000.

During his stay in Tampa, Dr. Nagamia received many distinctions and awards, including the Eisenhower Commission Award, the Distinguished Citizen Award from the City of Tampa, and the Distinguished Host and Model Citizen Award from the US Department of State. Among his own colleagues he gained great respect and was recognized with the Mother India International Award ("For Demonstrating Extraordinary Excellence in His Chosen Field"), as well as the Frederick A. Reddy MD Memorial Award for distinction as physician of the year and Distinguished Citizen recognition by the Hillsborough County Medical Association. Several of the hospitals where he was on staff honored him for his leadership and service, which he was always proud of. He was the author of many peer-reviewed papers on thoracic trauma and vascular diseases.

Dr. Nagamia's leadership qualities granted him professional membership in an assortment of well-known organizations. In 1973 he was awarded a fellowship from the International College of Surgeons. From 1980 to 1984 he was the editor in chief of the *Journal of the Islamic Medical Association* (JIMA). He was elected the president of the IMANA for 1984 and 1985.

Dr. Nagamia had a remarkable passion for Islam, Islamic history, and Islamic education. His quest for knowledge took him to many countries around the globe, including India, Pakistan, England, Spain, Turkey, South Africa, Malaysia, Saudi Arabia, and Egypt. He would take pictures and collect valuable books and relics, returning empowered by the glory of Islam. He would then reflect on them in his talks and publications.[1]

As an outcome of his passion, Dr. Nagamia oversaw the creation of an independent institution solely dedicated to Islamic medicine and science, and he became the founder of the International Institute of Islamic Medicine (IIIM) in 1992. For nearly three decades the institution was housed in Tampa under the banner of IMANA. In 2018 it was rededicated as the Nagamia Institute of Islamic Medicine and Science (NIIMS), the first of its kind in the United States. The institution was moved to the Rolling Meadows suburb of Chicago and housed in its own independent building. The mission statement of the organization said it well: "NIIMS acquires and disseminates knowledge of the rich history of Islamic Medicine and fosters its contemporary application." The vision statement defines it: "It is in the preservation and dissemination of knowledge and history that we aim to inspire excellence and action through faith." The institution values respect for all peoples, differences, and spiritual heritages. Besides researching the history of Islamic medicine, it has developed a Qur'an Museum that houses many unique and handwritten Qur'ans. Monthly educational webinars and teaching calligraphy have been established to impart knowledge on the history of Islamic medicine and its current advancements. Recently the board has expanded the vision and activities of the organization and, to be all inclusive, has renamed it as the Islamic Institute of Medicine Art and Culture (IIMAC).

Dr. Nagamia was also among the founders of many national organizations, including the ISNA, IMANA and the American Federation of Muslims of Indian Origin (AFMI), which is dedicated to universal education for minorities in India with a goal of achieving one-hundred percent literacy.

While living in Tampa, Dr. Nagamia and his family established many organizations and charities. They played a pivotal role in building the Islamic Society of Tampa Bay. The center has a large campus that includes a beautiful mosque, Islamic school, library, and food pantry. It functions as a place for youth activities, marriages, and funerals. He also started the Tampa Muslim Alliance, which promoted many yearly events like the Annual Muslim Charity Festival and an essay competition on the topic of the golden age of Islamic civilization. Doing so, laid the foundation for many interfaith relationships.

---

1. A short list of his publications is as follows: An Introduction to the History of Islamic Medicine; Prophetic Medicine: "A Holistic Approach to Medicine"; New Definition of Islamic Medicine: "Neo-Islamic Medicine"; A Museum and Library of Islamic Medical History: A New Perspective; The Great Physician Historian during the Golden Islamic Medical History: Ibn Abi Usaybi'aa; Abu Zayd Hunayn Ibn Ishaq al-Ibadi: A Physician Translator Par Excellence; The Bukhtishu Family: A Dynasty of Physicians in the Early History of Islamic Medicine; Islamic Medicine History and the Current Practice; and What Is Wrong with American Medicine? The Role of IMANA.

Throughout his life journey, Dr. Nagamia received dedicated companionship from his wife of fifty-five years, Dr. Zubeda Nagamia. She shared his passion and commitment and traveled the world with him. She was a practicing anesthesiologist in Tampa.

His daughter, Dr. Afshan Ahmed, is a dentist who graduated from Ohio State University and is married to Dr. Ashfaq Ahmed. They live in Springfield, Ohio, and have two children, Armaan Ahmed, studying at New York University, and Amin Ahmed, studying finance at the University of Pennsylvania. His son, Dr. Sameer Nagamia, is an interventional cardiologist practicing in Tampa.

Dr. Nagamia made Islam his way of life and his dedication and commitments were exemplary. He had the unique gift for effectively balancing his time between his profession, his Islamic work, and his community and family obligations. It will be a long time before we see another human being of his caliber. Dr. Nagamia reminds me of a couplet written by the great Islamic poet and philosopher Allama Iqbal:

Hazaron saal nargis apni be noori pe roti hay;
Bari mushkil se hota hay chaman mein deedawar payda

The narcissus (flower) has been lamenting its blindness for a thousand years;
How rare and difficult it is for anyone born in this garden to develop true vision.

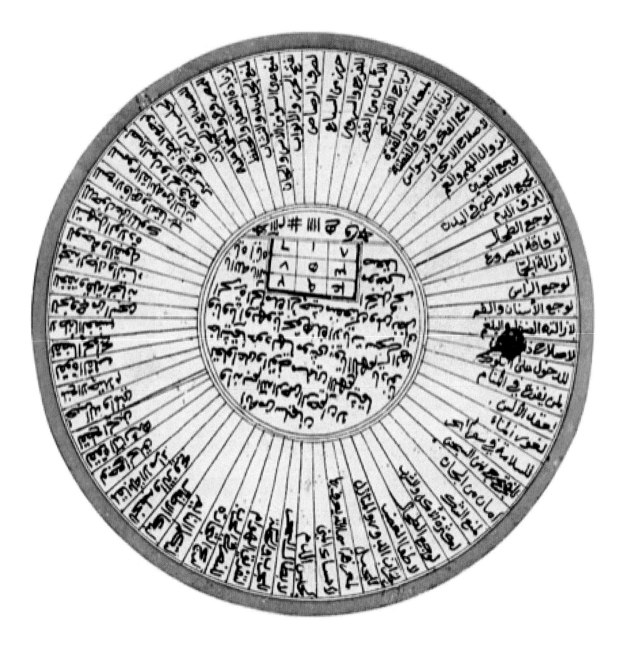

Curative Arabic Talisman used during the Golden Age of Islamic Civilization

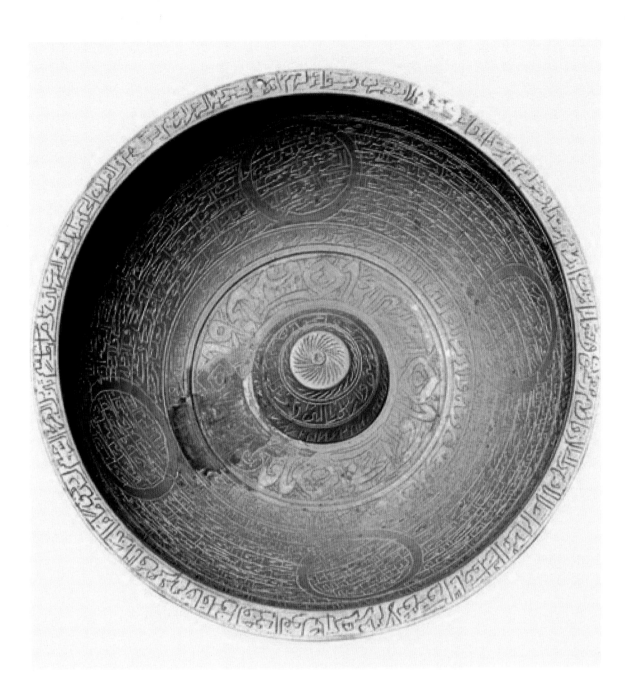

Copper bowl with Qur'anic calligraphy used for drinking water

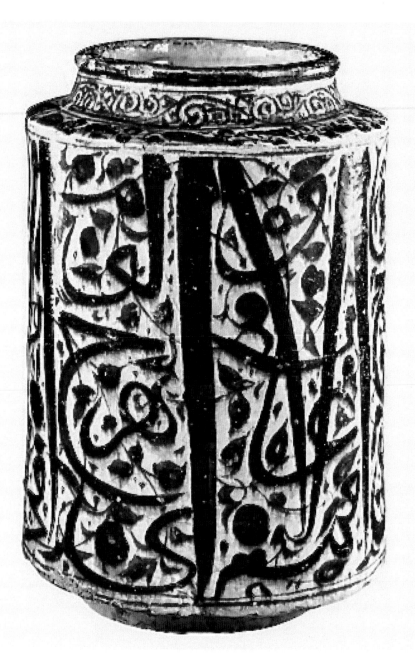

Medicine container with Qur'anic calligraphy

CHAPTER 2:

An Introduction to the History of Islamic Medicine

Husain Nagamia, MD, FRCS

Abstract

The development of medicine and other sciences during the Islamic era is not well documented by recent historians. Many modern books on the history of medicine devote only a cursory description to the period, and some bypass it entirely. Some historians even state that there were no notable advances made in medical science during the Islamic era from 642 CE to 1452 CE, when the decline and breakup of the Islamic empire started. Only in recent years, based on extensive fresh research historians concluded that medicine not only made great strides and advancements during the Islamic era, but the very basis of modern medicine was founded during this "golden" period. During this time, Muslim physicians gathered existing medical knowledge and texts from all the known parts of the Eastern world and from all the lands that Muslims eventually conquered and ruled. Medical knowledge came even from distant lands such as China and India, which were at the farthest regions of the Islamic empire. Having accumulated all this knowledge, it was systemized, analyzed, researched, and improved upon. The following article briefly examines this tantalizing period in the history of medicine, paying tribute to the physicians and scientists who laid the foundation for Islamic medicine. Many references have been appended at the end of the article for those who wish to undertake a further in-depth study of this fascinating subject.

Key Term: *history of Islamic medicine, medicine during the Islamic era, Arab medicine, prophetic medicine*

Considerable confusion exists in the literature regarding the definition of Islamic medicine. This is mainly because authors who write about Islamic medicine are writing about one aspect of it [1][2][3][4]. Thus, the definition can vary depending upon the perspective. The context can be historical, cultural, scientific, and pharmacologic, therapeutic, religious, or even geopolitical. In this monograph, we shall examine this body of knowledge, mainly from its historical, scientific, therapeutic, and application viewpoints.

The main source of all inspirational knowledge in Islam is the Holy Quran.[5] Muslims consider this book to have been revealed by God to Muhammad [PBUH]. "Aḥādīth" or "Sunnah,"[6] the recorded and authenticated sayings and traditions of what the Prophet Muhammad [PBUH] said and did, are a secondary source of a Muslim's inspiration.

Although the Qur'an is the guiding spirit that every Muslim follows, including physicians and their patients, Medicine per se is not mentioned much aside from a few comments concerning the beneficial effects of certain natural foods such as honey[7] and abstinence from drinking alcohol or other intoxicants.[8,9] However, very early in the Islamic era, the hadith literature accumulated a number of sayings and traditions of the Prophet [PBUH] under a collection called "Prophetic Medicine"[10] These edicts expounded on the virtues of right diet, natural remedies, and management of simple ailments such as headache, fever, sore throat, conjunctivitis, etc. More importantly, injunctions were given against contact with persons having contagious diseases, for instance leprosy, and against entering or leaving an area of an epidemic or plague, thus helping to limit the spread of a disease. In addition, many traditions were collected under the title of "spiritual medicine." These consisted of verses of the Qur'an or prayers to Allāh [SWT], which invoked blessings, and which were to be recited to relieve an affliction.

Prophetic Medicine

"Prophetic medicine," although popular among the masses due to its doctrinal and theological contexts, was considered by most Muslim historians and physicians as distinct from scientific and analytical Islamic medicine. Ibn Khaldūn (1332–1406 CE), the well-known medieval Muslim jurist, historian, and statesman, in his al-Muqaddimah[10] states: "The Bedouins in their culture, have a kind of medicine which they base primarily on experience restricted to a few patients only, and which they have inherited from their tribal leaders and elder

1. Rahman F: Health and medicine in the Islamic tradition. Crossroad Publishing Co. New York, 1987.
2. Brown EG: Arabian medicine. Cambridge University Press, Cambridge, 1962.
3. Ullman M: Islamic medicine. Edinburgh University Press, Edinburgh, 1978.
4. Rosenthal F: Science and medicine in Islam. Variorum. Hampshire, United Kingdom, 1990.
5. Abdullah Yūsuf 'Alī, The Holy Qur'ān, text and translation and commentary. Amana Corporation, Brentwood, MD, 1989.
6. Saḥīḥ al-Bukhārī.
7. Glorious Qur'ān, chapter 16, verse 69.
8. Glorious Qur'ān, chapter 2, verse 219.
9. Glorious Qur'ān, chapter 5, verse 90.
10. Al-Akili M: Natural healing with the medicine of the Prophet. Pearl Publishing, Philadelphia, 1993.
*Subhanahu wa taa'lah (SWT).

women. In some cases, it is effective, but it is not founded on natural laws, nor is it tested against (scientific accounts)."

Definition

Islamic medicine in its true context can be defined as a body of medical knowledge inherited by Muslims during the early phase of Islamic history (40–247 AH/661–861 CE) mostly from Greek sources to which knowledge from Persia, Syria, India, and Byzantium was added. This knowledge was not only translated into Arabic, the literary and scientific lingua franca of the time, but was also expounded, assimilated, exhaustively added to, and subsequently codified, and "Islamized." The physicians of the times, both Muslim and non-Muslim, added to this their own observations and experimentation, transforming it into a flourishing and practical science, helping to not only curing the ailments of the masses and increasing their standard of health. The effects of its dominating influence extended not only across the vast stretch of the Islamic lands, but also reached adjoining regions of Europe, Asia, China, and the Far East. It was measurable for an entire millennium, from the seventh to the seventeenth century CE, during which time, Europe was in the grips of the "dark ages." It set the standard for hygiene and preventative medicine and improved the general health of the masses globally. It was to hold sway until the political decline of the Islamic empire. With the advent of the European Renaissance, at the beginning of the 17th century CE, Islamic medicine was finally challenged by the newly emerging science of modern medicine, which finally replaced it in most of the countries, including the countries of its birth.

Historical Background

To understand the milieu in which Islamic medicine was born, one has to understand the salient events in the advent of Islam and a few events just preceding the Islamic era. The nomadic tribe of Bedouins roamed Arabia, which was a large area covered mostly by an arid desert. Certain communities had been established along trade routes, intersections and where water was available. Mecca was along the Yemen-Damascus trade route. It was considered a holy city and a sanctuary. The "Ka'abah," or house of worship, was replete with idols of different gods, each representing a tribe or community. These Bedouins had their own tribal moral or ethical codes of conduct, and idolatry, the worship of idols, was in practice. Blood feuds were common, and attacking caravans along the trade route was a way of life. Sacrifices often were offered to appease the gods; burying of live female children was common practice. Family feuds were common, and settling scores to uphold tribal honor led to frequent bloody encounters in which many people were killed. Women and children were treated as "chattels," or private possessions, and became the property of the winner. This era of Arabia is frequently referred by Muslims as "al-Jāhiliyyah" (the age of ignorance).

Islam not only brought dramatic changes in the religious practices of these warring nomadic tribes but also served to unite them into an unprecedented social and cultural nation that very quickly developed into a strong political entity with its own system of administration, justice, and military power. The first leader of the Islamic state was of course the Prophet of Islam, Muhammad [PBUH]. His four successors, called the Pious or "rightly guided" Caliphs, quickly expanded and consolidated its territories. Within about 100 years the Islamic empire had spread from Spain in the west to China in the east, encompassing western India as well. Later, it would be carried even farther by the Muslim merchants to the Malaysian peninsula, the islands of the East Indies, and Indonesia. In its early era and continuing for several centuries, the Islamic empire was ruled by a single leader or caliph and administered by provincial governors. The first four caliphs were elected democratically, later the caliphate became dynastic. A relatively separate "western caliphate" was established in Spain. Gradually, this geographically extensive Islamic empire would break up into various kingdoms, as its provincial rulers became more autonomous and independent. Ultimately, extensive portions were re-united by the Seljuk Turks, the forerunners of the Ottoman Empire.

It was during the early caliphates of the Umayyads and the Abbasids that the main development of Islamic medicine took place. It was also during this time and under the patronage of these caliphs that across the Islamic lands the great physicians, both Muslim and non-Muslim, thrived accumulating the wealth of medical knowledge and cultivating a system of medicine that was later called "Islamic medicine."

The early era of Islamic medicine and the school of medicine at Jundishapur or "Gondeshapur" was a city in Khuzistan founded by a Sassanid emperor, Shapur I (247–272 CE) before the advent of Islam. In present day western Persia, the site is marked by the ruins of Shahabad near the city of Ahwāz. The town was taken by Muslims during the caliphate of Hazrat 'Umar, the second guided caliph, by 'Abū Mūsā al-'Ashari in (17 AH/738 CE). At this time, it already had a well-established hospital and medical school. Many Syrians took refuge in the city when Shapur I captured Antioch. In fact, Shapur I nicknamed the city "Vehaz-Andevi Shaput" (Shapur is better than Antioch). The closing of the Nestorian School of Edessa by Emperor Zeno in 489 CE led to the Nestorians fleeing from there and seeking refuge in Jundishapur under patronage of Shapur II, which got an academic boost as a result. The Greek influence was already predominant in Jundishapur when the closing of the Athenian academy in 529 CE by order of the Byzantine emperor Justanian drove many learned Greek physicians to this town. A university with a medical school and a hospital was established by Khosrow Anushirwan the Wise (531–571 CE), and Greco-Syrian medicine blossomed. To this was added medical knowledge from India brought by the physician "Burzuyah," the vizier of Anushirwan. On his return, he brought back from India the famous "Fables of Bidpai," several Indian physicians' details of Indian medical tests and a Pahlavi translation of the "Kalīlah and Dimnah," Mirror for Princes. Khosrow was even presented with a translation of Aristotelian logic and philosophy. Thus, at the time of the Islamic invasion, the school of Jundishapur was well established and had become renowned as a medical center of Greek, Syrian, and Indian learning. This knowledge had intermingled to create a highly acclaimed and state-of-the-art medical school and hospital. After the advent of Islamic rule, the university continued to thrive. In fact, the first recorded Muslim physician, Harīth ibn-Kaladah, who was a contemporary of the Prophet [PBUH], acquired his medical knowledge at this medical school and hospital in Jundishapur.

It is likely that the medical teaching at Jundishapur was modeled after the teachings at Alexandria with some influence from Antioch, but it is important to note that the treatment was based entirely on scientific analysis in true Hippocratic tradition, rather than a combination of superstition and ritual, as was the case in Greek "asclepieia" and Byzantine "nosocomia." This hospital and medical center were to become the model from which all later Islamic medical schools and hospitals were to be built. The school thrived during the

Umayyad caliphate, and Sergus of Rasul'in translated medical and philosophical works of both Hippocrates and Galen into Syrian. These were later translated into Arabic, casting an everlasting imprint onto the future of Islamic medicine.

It was during the Abbasid caliphate that Caliph al-Mansūr, the founder of the city of Baghdad, invited the then head of the Jundishapur School to treat him. This physician was Jirjis Bukhtyishu, a Christian whose name meant "Jesus has saved." He treated the caliph successfully and was appointed to the court. He, however, did not stay in Baghdad permanently, instead returning to Jundishapur before his death. The migration to Baghdad had begun. Thus, his son Jibril Bukhtishu established a practice in the city and became a prominent physician. Another family that migrated from Jundishapur to Baghdad was the family of Māsawīh who came at the invitation of Caliph Harun-al-Rashid. Māsawīh became a famous ophthalmologist. Most famous among his three sons who were physicians was Yūhanna ibn Māsawīh (Mesue Senior). He wrote prolifically, and 42 works were attributed to him. By this time second half of the 2nd century after 'Hijrah, the Prophet's migration to Medina (8th century CE), the fame of Baghdad began to rise as also the political power of the caliphate. Many hospitals and medical centers were established, and tremendous intellectual activity was recorded. This culminated into the period of Islamic Renaissance and the golden era of Islamic medicine which will be covered under a separate section.

The Resources for Development of Islamic Medicine

"Bait-ul-Hikmah," or the House of Wisdom

It was founded in 214 AH/830 CE by the Caliph al-Ma'mūn, an Abbasid caliph ibn al-Nadīm, who was the son of a bookseller and whose famous catalog of books, "Fihrist of Nadīm," tells us of many of the books of his time and relates this story of the caliph: Aristotle appeared in the dream of the learned caliph and told him that there was no conflict between reason and revelation. The caliph thus set about searching for books and manuscripts of the ancient Greek philosophers and scientists. He sent an emissary to the Byzantine emperor to get all the scientific manuscripts that were apparently stored in an old and dilapidated building. After initially turning down his request, the emperor granted it. Among the emissaries sent to select the work was the first director of the House of Wisdom, Salman, who was the one who led the delegation. Others in it were al-Hajjāj ibn Matar and ibn al-Batrīq. They brought back with them many Greek scientific works and manuscripts. Translations of all of these were immediately started. However, the translation of the medical works of the Greeks had started earlier during the reign of Caliph Hārūn al-Rashīd, with the building of the first hospital under the caliph's patronage. Ibn al-Nadim lists 57 translations associated with the House of Wisdom. The translators who formed the first delegation to the Byzantine king have already been named. Famous translations are as follows:

1. Al-Hajjāj ibn Yusuf ibn Matar completed a translation of Euclid's elements. Other Greek authors including Aristotle, Archimedes, Pythagoras, Theodosius, Jerash, Apollonius, Theron, and Menelaus all were translated.

2. Muhammad ibn Mūsā al-Khawarizmi systematically explored arithmetic and algebra. The latter derived its name from his discourse, "Kitāb al-Jabr wāl-Muqābalah." Algebra was derived from the second letter and meant "bone setting," a graphic description of operations on solving quadratic equations.

3. The knowledge of geometry flourished, and with-it architecture and design. Ibn Khaldūn was later to describe geometry as a science that "enlightens the intelligence of man and cultivates rational thinking."

4. Al-Ma'mūn's court astronomer was Mūsā ibn Shākir. His three sons, Muhammad, Ahmad, and al-Hasan devoted their lives to the search of knowledge. They exemplified the Prophetic traditions and dicta "Seek learning even if it be in China." "The search for knowledge is obligatory on every Muslim." As a popular saying goes: "The ink of scholars is worth more than the blood of martyrs."

5. The works of these learned men, or "Sons of Mūsā (Moses)," were exceptionally creative. They wrote on celestial mechanics, the atom, the origins of the earth, Ptolemaic universe, the properties of the ellipse, plane, and spheres. The knowledge of geometry served in practice to create canals, bridges, and architectural designs.

6. Muhammad ibn Mūsā on one of his travels met Thābit ibn Qurrah. The latter was master in three languages—Greek, Syrian, and Arabic—and soon got appointed to become the court astrologer to caliph al-Mu'tadid. He was an invaluable addition to the House of Wisdom. In 70 original works, he wrote on every conceivable subject, including mathematics, astronomy, astrology, ethics, mechanics, physics, philosophy, and published commentaries on Euclid, Ptolemy, and other famous Greek thinkers and philosophers.

7. The two sons of Thābit ibn Qurrah also became famous. Sinān was a famous physician in Baghdad. He was director of several hospitals and was court physician to three successive caliphs. His son Ibrāhīm also became a prominent scientist. He invented sundials and wrote a special treatise on this subject.

8. The greatest medical mind in the House of Wisdom was Hunayn ibn Ishāq. Born in Hua, Hunayn was the son of a pharmacist(apothecary). He soon translated the entire collection of Greek medical works, including Galen and Hippocrates. Hunayn was an extremely gifted and talented translator. As being just a literal translator, he tended to be more scientific and duly interpreted the original text by cross references, annotation, and citing glossaries. His original contribution included 10 works on ophthalmology, which were extremely systematic. He rose to the highest honor by being appointed the director of the House of Wisdom by Caliph al-Mutawakkil.

9. Qūsta ibn Lūqā was another accomplished translator and scholar. He had 40 original contributions to his credit. He wrote on the diverse subjects such as mirrors, hairs, fans, winds, logic, geometry, and astronomy.

10. Yuhannā ibn Māsawīh (Mesue Senior) was an early director of the House of Wisdom. He served under four caliphs: al-Ma'mūn, al-Mu'tasim, al Wathiq, and al-Mutawakkil. He wrote about medical, especially gynecologic, problems.

11. The effect of the House of Wisdom was tremendous. Islamic science, philosophy, art, and architecture all felt its effects. Agriculture, government, prosperity, and economic wealth were the benefactors. It ultimately was responsible for producing figures such as al-Kindī, al-Fārabī, some of the greatest thinkers, scientists, and philosophers of Islam. Also, some of the greatest Islamic physicians had available to them all the knowledge of ancient Greece, Syria, India, and Persia. In turn, they contributed by their astute observation and originality. The giants of Islamic medicine and their achievements are described elsewhere in this chapter.

Hospitals during the Islamic Era

The idea of a hospital as an institutional place for the caring of the sick had not existed in antiquity. There were sanatoria and "travel lodges" that were attached to temples where attendant priests looked after the sick. Most of the therapy in these sanatoria consisted of prayers and sacrifices to the gods of healing, especially to Aesculapius. Cures that occurred were thought to result from divine intervention.

Many hospitals were developed early during the Islamic era. They were to be called "bimāristān" (place for the sick) or "māristān." The idea of a hospital as a place where the sick could get attention was totally adopted by the early caliphs. The first hospital is credited to Caliph al-Walīd I, an Umayyad caliph (86–96 AH/705–715 CE). To some, however, it was considered no more than a leprosarium because it allowed segregation of lepers from others. It had salaried doctors on staff to attend to the sick.

The first true Islamic hospital was built during the reign of Caliph Harun-al-Rashid (170–193 AH/786–809 CE). Having heard of the famous medical institution at Jundishapur, already described above, the caliph invited the son of the chief physician Jibril Bakhtishu to come to Baghdad to head the new bimāristān, which he did. It rapidly achieved fame and led quickly to the development of other hospitals in Baghdad. One of these "audidi" hospitals was to be built under the instruction of the great Islamic physician al-Rāzī. It is said that to select the best site for the hospital he had pieces of meat hung in various quarters of the city and watched their putrefaction. He advised the caliph to put the hospital where the putrefaction was the slowest and least. At its inception, this hospital had 24 physicians on staff, including a specialist categorized as a physiologist, oculists, surgeons, and bonesetters. Djubīr visited Baghdad in 580 AH/1184 CE and reported that this hospital was "like a great castle" with a water supply from the Tigris and all appurtenances of royal palaces.

1. One of the largest and most elaborate hospitals ever built was the Mansūri Hospital in Cairo. It was completed in 1248 CE by the order of the Mameluke ruler of Egypt, Mansūr Qalāwūn. It could hold 8,000 people. The annual income from endowments alone was one million dirhams. Men and women were admitted to separate wards. Irrespective of race, religion, creed, or citizenship (as specifically stated in the waqf documents) nobody was turned away. There was not a limit on the times the patient was treated as an inpatient (a contrast to today's HMOs). There were separate wards for men and women, and medicine, surgery, fevers, and

eye disease had separate wards. It had its own pharmacy, library, and lecture halls. It had a mosque for Muslim patients as well as a chapel for Christian patients. The waqf document, an endowment made by a Muslim to a religious, educational, or charitable cause specifically stated:

> "The hospital shall keep all patients, men, and women, until they are completely recovered. All costs are to be borne by the hospital whether the people come from afar or near. Whether they are resident or foreigners, strong or weak, low, or high, rich or poor, employed or unemployed, blind or sighted, physically or mentally ill, learned or illiterate. There are no conditions of consideration for payment, none is objected to or even indirectly hunted at for nonpayment. The entire service is through the magnificent of Allāh, the generous one."

As to the physical condition of these hospitals, especially those established by princes, rulers, and viziers, some were luxurious and were actual palaces that had been converted to hospitals. Even contemporary Europe could not boast of a single hospital that came close to the facilities that were provided in these institutions. Some of these, especially in Baghdad, Egypt, and Syria, had furnishings that were like those in the palaces. Most of these being under the patronage of the viziers, sultans, and caliphs were no doubt inspired by the Islamic teaching of the welfare of the poor and needy. The Qur'ān tells us: "You shall not attend to virtue unless you spend for the welfare of poor from the choicest part of your wealth."

And again: "You who believe spend (for the poor) from the worthiest part of what you have earned and what your crop yields, and do not give away from its unworthy parts such that you yourselves will not take until you examine the quality minutely—and know that Allāh is not in your need and all praise belongs to Him."[11]

As to the salaries of physicians, here is some information from authentic sources. The annual income of Jibrīl ibn Bakhitshu, who was the chief of staff at a Baghdad hospital during the reign of Ma'mūn al-Rashīd, as recorded by his own secretary, was 4.9 million dirhams. His son, also a doctor, lived in a house in Baghdad that was air conditioned by ice in summer and heated by charcoal in winter. A resident, by comparison, was supposed to be on duty for two days and two nights a week and was paid 300 dirhams a month. (Remind you of Denton Cooley and his fellows?)

The Great Physicians of Islamic Medicine

The era of Islamic medicine produced some famous and notable physicians. These physicians were not only responsible for gathering all the existing information on medicine of the time but also for adding their own astute observation, experimentation, and skills. Many of them were skilled in medical writing and produced encyclopedic works, which became standard texts and reference works for centuries. With the coming of the European Renaissance, they formed the basis on which the European authors gained insight into the medicine of the "ancient," or early Greek authors, whose works were only preserved in Arabic. In addition, many rediscoveries took place, which had already been recorded by Islamic physicians but hitherto had been unknown until

---

11. Goodman LE: Avicenna Routledge Publications. London and New York, 1992.

recently uncovered. The classic example of the discovery of pulmonary circulation originally given to Servetus, was found to have been succinctly described by ibn al-Nafis, an Islamic physician who lived centuries earlier. Ibn al-Nafis repudiated the earlier concepts held by Galen and described the lesser circulation so succinctly that nothing more could be added until Malphigi could describe the alveoli and pulmonary capillaries with the advent of the microscope discovered by Antonie van Leeuwenhoek in the mid 17th century. Some of them form the basis of instruction of students of al-Tibb and al-Hikmah, the traditional Islamic medicine practiced in the subcontinent of India and Pakistan, even today under the banner of Tibb or Yūnāni medicine. It would be out of scope for us in this article to describe the accomplishments of each of these physicians., However, here we will proceed with giving you the salient accomplishments of some of the most notable among them. For the sake of classification, the history period of Islamic physician can be divided into three parts:

1. The period of the Islamic Renaissance, from the beginning of Islamic to the end of the Abbasid dynasty.

2. The period of the Islamic epoch, when all science, including medicine, reached the pinnacle of development under the Islamic patronage.

3. The period of decline, during which the knowledge of Islamic medicine was translated into European languages and became the basis for further development and discoveries and ultimately led to the development of modern medicine.

The Period of the Islamic Renaissance

The notable physicians during this period are as follows:

1. The Bukhtishu family of physicians. The oldest amongst these was Jibril Bukhtishu, who was the chief physician at the hospital in Jundishapur. He came from a Christian family and was summoned to the court of Caliph Ma'mūn (148 AH/765 CE), where the latter fell ill. After having treated him successfully, he was invited to stay in Baghdad and head a hospital there. He declined and returned to his native Jundishapur (152AH/769 CE). It was his son Jirjis Bukhtishu who was later invited by Caliph Hārūn-al-Rashid to come to Baghdad to treat him (171 AH/787 CE) and was then offered to be the chief physician and head a hospital in Baghdad, which he did until he died in 185 AH/801 CE.

2. Māsawīh is another family of physicians associated with early Islamic history. During the reign of Caliph Hārūn-al-Rashid, the elder of the family migrated from Jundishapur to Baghdad and became a celebrated ophthalmologist. He wrote the first Arabic treatise on ophthalmology. His son, known to the west as Mesue Senior and whose name is Yūhannā ibn Māsawīh, wrote several medical works in Arabic while translating other works from Greek. He is known for having somewhat of a sarcastic temperament; nevertheless, he commanded great respect because of his medical expertise.

3. Hunayn ibn Ishāq, a student of ibn Māsawīh's, became the greatest translator of Greek and Syriac medical texts during the 3rd century AH/9th CE. He was responsible for the masterly translations

from Classical Greek into Arabic, of Galen, Hippocrates, and Aristotle. He also improved the Arabic medical lexicon, giving it a rich technical language to express medical terminology and laid the foundation of a rich medical expression in the Arabic language, far exceeding the later translation from Arabic to Latin. He was an astute physician and wrote two original works on ophthalmology.

The credit for the first systematic work on medicine during this era goes to a Muslim physician, Alī ibn Rabbān al Tabbāri, hailing from Persia but settling in Baghdad in the first half of the 3rd century AH/9th century CE. His work called "Firdūs al-Hikmah" (Paradise of Wisdom) contained extensive medical information from all extant sources including Greek, Syria, Persian, and Indian and contained an extensive treatment of anatomy.

The Period of the Islamic Epoch

Perhaps the most famous and notable physician, perhaps of the entire early Islamic era is Muhammad ibn Zakariyyā al-Rāzī (born 251 AH/865 CE, died 312 AH/925 CE), also known by his Latinized name Rhazes. Other than his birthplace in Rayy in northern Persia, not much is known about his early life or his medical education. His fame starts with the establishment of a hospital in Baghdad of which he was the chief. The story of how he picked the site of the hospital has become one of the classic legends of Islamic medicine. He suspended pieces of meat in various quarters of the city and examined them later for putrefaction. He recommended the site where the meat had decayed the least as the most suitable site, thus making him the first physician to infer indirectly the bacteriological putrefaction of meat and the environmental role that the contamination of air played in the spread of infection, predating by centuries the modern concept of airborne infection.

Besides this astute observation, al-Rāzī is known for numerous other original contributions to the arts and the science of medicine. Although not the first to describe the difference between smallpox and chicken-pox and provide a detailed description of measles in his famous work "Kitab al Judarī wa 'l hasbah" (Treatise on Smallpox and Measles), this work became well known in the West because of its frequent translation. He described allergy to roses in one of his classical cases. The famous Islamic historian and scientist al-Birūnī has listed 56 medical works of al-Rāzi, the best-known being "Kitab al-Hāwī fi al-Tibb or "The Comprehensive Book of Medicine," an encyclopedia of medical knowledge based on his personal observations and experiences. A scribal copy of this book was recently exhibited by the National Library of Medicine in Bethesda, Maryland, celebrating the 900th anniversary of its completion. The copy is by an unknown scribe and has been recorded as the third oldest medical manuscript preserved in the world today. (A shorter medical textbook was dedicated to Caliph al-Mansūr and hence called "Kitāb al-Mansūrī.")

Besides these and other original contributions, of which most have been published, and some survive to this day, al-Rāzi devoted a lot of his time to teaching, bedside medicine, and attending to the royalty and court. The impact of his publications on Islamic medicine was tremendous. His books became an invaluable addition to the armaments of a medical student of the time and remained the standard text until the appearance much later of texts by al-Majūsī (see below) and ibn Sina's "Al-Qānun fil Tibb" (The Canon of Medicine) of which descriptions will be given later.

In the 4th century of hijra, 10th century CE, another Islamic physician gained prominence in Baghdad. His name was al-Majūsī or known as Haly Abbas in the West (d. 384 AH/994 CE). He became the director of the Adud al-Dawlah hospital. It was to its founder that al-Majūsī dedicated his medical work entitled "Kitāb Kāmil al-Sinā ah al-Tibbiyah" (The Complete Book of Medical Art), also called "al-Kitāb al-Malaki" (The Royal Book). This book (of which again a copy is preserved in the National Library of Medicine at Bethesda) is very well systematized and organized. It is divided into two basic volumes, of which one covers theory, and one covers the other practical aspects. Each of these volumes has 10 chapters. The first volume deals with historical sources, anatomy, faculties, six primeval functions, classifications, and causation of disease, and internal disease such as fever, headache, epilepsy, and warning signs of death or recovery. The second volume deals with hygiene, diet, cosmetics, therapy with simple drugs, therapy for fevers and disease or organs viz of respiration, digestion, reproduction, etc. There is a chapter on surgery, another orthopedics, and, finally, treatment by compound medicines.

About the 2nd century AH/8th century AD, a great center of knowledge, learning, and culture was already developing in the western part of the Islamic empire in Spain, or the "Andalus," as it was called by the Arabs. Spain had been invaded and conquered by the Muslims in 93 AH/714 CE. When the Umayyad dynasty ended in Baghdad, the last of the Umayyad princes escaped to Spain, where they established a great dynasty called the Western Caliphate. The rulers of this dynasty laid the foundation of the Muslim rule of Spain that was to last seven centuries. The advent of this period occurred during the reign of Amir 'Abdul-Rahmān al-Dakhīl (Abd al-Rahman I ibn Mu'awiya) around AH 138 756 CE. During his reign (756-788 CE) Cordoba, or Qurtubah, became a great center of international learning. In the next two centuries, a library containing more than one million volumes was established, sciences flourished, and scholars and physicians worked under the royal patronage of 'Abdul-Rahmān III al Nāsir (AH 300–350/ 912/961 CE).

Perhaps the most famous physician and surgeon of the Umayyad age in Spain was 'Abū al-Qāsim Khalaf ibn al-Abbās al-Zahrāwī, known to the West as Albucasis (AH 318-403/ 930-1013 CE). He gained great fame as a physician and wrote a major compendium of extant medical knowledge entitled "al-Tasrif." It comprised 30 volumes. The initial volumes dealt with general principles, the elements and physiology of humors, the rest dealt with the systematic treatment of disease, from the head to the feet. The last volume is perhaps the most important in that it dealt with all aspects of surgery. It was the first textbook of surgery to be published with illustrations of the instruments used. It gained such great fame that it became the standard textbook of surgery in important universities in Christian Europe and was widely read. Al-Zahrāwī emphasized that a knowledge of anatomy and physiology was essential prior to undertaking any surgery. He said:

"Before practicing surgery, he (the surgeon) should gain knowledge of anatomy and the function of organs so that he will understand their shape, connections, and borders. He should become thoroughly familiar with nerves, muscles, bones, arteries, and veins. If one does not comprehend anatomy and physiology, one can commit a mistake which will result in the death of the patient. I have seen someone incise into a swelling on the neck thinking it was an abscess, when it was an aneurysm, and the patient died on the spot."

Some operations described by him are carried out today in the manner he described 1000 years ago. These include operations on varicose veins, the reduction of skull fractures, dental extractions, and the forceps delivery of a dead fetus, to mention just a few. Surgery was raised by al-Zahrāwī to the level of a high science at a time when the Council of Tours in Europe declared in 1163 CE.: "Surgery is to be abandoned by all schools of medicine and by all decent physicians."

Another man widely regarded as the greatest physician of the classical Islamic era was Avicenna, or 'Abū 'Ali al-Husain ibn 'Abdullah ibn Sinā. Some historians of medicine acclaim him as the greatest physician ever. This is perhaps because ibn Sina was not only a physician par excellence, but also because he possessed knowledge and wisdom that extended to many other branches of science and culture, including philosophy, metaphysics, logic, and religion. As a result of his great wisdom, he was awarded the titles al-Sheikh, al-Ra'īs (the chief master), and al-Mu'allim al-Thānī (the second philosopher, after Aristotle).

Ibn Sīnā was indeed a prodigy. At the age of 10, he had memorized the whole Qur'an. By the age of 16, he had mastered all extant sciences that appealed to him, including mathematics, geometry, Islamic law, logic, philosophy, and metaphysics. By 18, he had taught himself all that there was to learn in medicine. Born in the city of Bukhārā, in what is now Uzbekistan, in 370 AH/980 CE, he rapidly showed enough ability to become the vizier and court physician of the city's Samanid ruler, Prince Nūh ibn Mansūr. The royal library was opened to him, and this took his knowledge into new dimensions. He began writing his first book at 21. In the short span of 30 years, he wrote more than 100 books, of which 16 were on medicine. The "Canon of Medicine," as it became known in the West, was entitled of "Kitāb al-Qānūn fil Tibb." This voluminous compendium of medical knowledge rivaled the efforts of al-Rāzi and al-Majūsi, and indeed surpassed them in content and originality. It was composed of five volumes: Volume I contained general principles; Volume II, simple drugs; Volume III, a systematic description of diseases from head to foot; Volume IV, general maladies, viz fevers; and Volume V, compound drugs. The Canon was translated into Latin by Gerard of Cremona and Andrea Alpago in Toledo. It remained the standard textbook of medicine in Louvain and Montpellier until the 17th century. A complete copy exists in the archives of the National Library of Medicine in Bethesda, Maryland. [12] The effects of the systematic collection of hitherto unorganized Greco-Roman medicine, and the addition of ibn Sīnā's personal observation and experimentation, brought medicine to a new pinnacle of excellence.

Writes Emile Savage Smith, professor of history at the Wellcome Library of Medicine, in a monograph that accompanied an exhibition of the oldest Arabic manuscripts in a collection at the National Library of Medicine: "The medicine of the day was so brilliantly clarified by these compendia (especially those of ibn Sina and al-Majūsi) and such order and consistency was brought to it that a sense of perfection and hence stultifying authority resulted."[12][13]

The Basic Sciences in Islamic Medicine

Contrary to popular belief, basic sciences were highly developed in the lands of Islam. For instance, Oriental historians of medicine have erroneously suggested that the science of anatomy during the Islamic era was rudimentary and did not progress much further than the discoveries already made and described by the Greeks,

---

12. The first three books in Arabic are viewable on-line at https://www.loc.gov/resource/gdcwl.wdl 15431/?st=gallery
13. Savage-Smith E: Islamic culture and medical arts. National Library of Medicine. Bethesda, MD, 1994.

or "the ancients." It was popularly held that Islamic physicians did not challenge the anatomic concepts of the "ancients," partly because of the "religious proscription" against dissection, and thus, lacking in their own observations, they relied heavily on the observations of Galen, Aristotle, Paul of Agaeia, and other Greek sources. However, after recent discoveries of manuscripts by an Egyptian physician, Muhyīl-dīn al-Tatāwī, which had not been hitherto scrutinized, Islamic physicians not only possessed an excellent knowledge of anatomy, but that they added some challenging new concepts that were revolutionary to the understanding in their day of the anatomical concepts laid down by the Greeks. One now well-known example is the discovery of the lesser or pulmonary circulation by ibn al-Nafīs (d 687AH/1288 CE), who suggested that there existed a pulmonary capillary bed where the blood was "purified" before being brought back to the heart by the pulmonary artery. Until then, credit for the discovery of the lesser, or pulmonary, circulation was given to the Spaniard Servetus and the Italian Colombo, who independently described it in very similar to ibn al-Nafīs, only 200 years later. The description given of the pulmonary circulation by ibn al-Nafīs challenged the fundamental concept held by Galen, predating by 400 years the discovery of pulmonary capillaries, following Anthony von Leuwenhoek's invention of the microscope in about 1668. It ought also to be mentioned that ibn Māsawīh, known in the west as Massue the Elder, had built, with the special permission of the caliph, a house on the banks of the Tigris where he dissected apes to learn their anatomy. He extrapolated from those results what information he could that might shed light on human anatomy. Al-Zahrāwī, in the surgical section of this book entitled al-Tasrif, offers this comment on anatomy:

> "Now this is the reason why there is no skillful surgeon in our day: the art of medicine is long and it is necessary for its exponent, before he exercises it, to be trained in anatomy as Galen has described it, so that he may be fully acquainted with the uses, forms, temperament of the limbs; also how they are jointed, and how they may be separated, that he should understand fully also the bones, tendons and muscles, their numbers and their attachments; and also the blood vessels, both the arteries and the veins, with their relations. And so, Hippocrates said: 'Though many are doctors in name, few in reality, particularly on the surgical side.'"

Regarding the physiologic concepts embodied in Islamic medicine, they were based on the Hippocratic and Galenical concepts of elements, natures, and humors, in which earth, fire, air, and water are each given a temperament: earth is dry and cold; water is humid and cold; fire is hot and dry heat; and air is humid and hot. Each of the four essential body fluids: blood, phlegm, yellow bile, and black bile, is assigned a respective temperament. Each dietary food, medicine, or climatic environment can thus modify or temper the humors of the body, and it is an interplay of these that can restore health from sickness or cause the sickness to worsen. According to this approach, harmony in the body prevails when all the humors are in proper balance, and it is their imbalance that creates disease, requiring a restoration of the body's natural balance. In conventional modern medicine such a concept would be unacceptable, or least untenable because the causation of disease is related to etiologic agents or factors. However, Claud Bernard's concept of the "milieu interior" can in modern terms be compared to the Jabirean concept of innate harmony, as expounded by Islamic medicine.

Such a theory was understandably rejected by western scientists although more recently scientists have begun to view the human body in a different light. Acupuncture is a good example. Until recently, the theoretical basis of acupuncture would not have been acceptable to any physician trained by principles of Western or modern medicine. Yet today, many physicians consider it acceptable, because the application has shown practical results. For a further exploration of the theories of Islamic medicine, the reader is directed to an exposition by OC Gruner, [14] and a dissertation on this subject by Hakīm Muhammad Sa'id.

More important, is the fundamental belief of a Muslim physician that the organic body alone cannot manifest life, it being in and of itself inanimate and devoid of a life force., and that it is the instillation of this life force, or "al-Rūh" (the spirit or soul), which gives the body its vibrancy and vitality. Without the Rūh, no function of the body is possible. It is the Rūh that descends, in a sense, from the Almighty to mix with the anatomic and physiologic body to make a complete human being. It is thus essential when treating a diseased state to take into consideration the Rūh, or soul, a concept alien to modern medicine.

Pharmacy, Pharmacognosy, Materia Medica, and Therapeutics

The development of pharmacy and pharmacognosy had a powerful influence on Islamic medicine. Most Islamic physicians and scholars studied chemistry or alchemy. Their study was furthered by the concomitant development of new techniques used to refine drugs, medications, and extracts by a process of distillation, sublimation, and crystallization. Druggists, or *attarin*, became commonplace in Islamic lands and their proliferation ultimately required the licensure of pharmacists and druggists.

Pharmacologic drugs were classified as simple and compound drugs, the "Mufradāt" and the "Murakkabāt." The effects of these two classes were detailed and documented. The earliest Islamic works on pharmacognosy were written before the translation of the influential ancient Greek works of Discorides (40 CE to 90 CE). Titles such as "Treatise on the Power of Drugs Their Beneficial and Their Ill Effects" and "The Power of Simple Drugs" were written in the 3rd and 4th century AH/9th century AD. Most medical texts contained chapters on the use of both these types of remedies. Al-Rāzī's al Hāwi mentions 829 drugs.

Materia Medica and texts containing compendia of drugs and their effects appear frequently during the era of Islamic medicine. Notable among these is the contribution of 'Abu Bakr Ibn Samghun of Cordoba. The second book of Ibn Sina's Canon is devoted to the discussion of simple drugs with their powers and qualities listed in charts. One of the most authoritative books on drugs was written by the scholar and philosopher, al-Bīrūni, entitled: "*The Book on Drugs*," which contains a huge compendium of drugs, their actions, and their equivalent names in several languages.

Even today, perhaps the most extensive pharmacotherapy, especially as related to plant medicinal and herbal preparations, may be attributed to modern-day Islamic or Tibbi medicine and finds great favor in the Indian subcontinent, often begin as popular as Western or allopathic medicines. Western pharmaceutical companies have often "invaded" this domain, the classical example being the extract of Ruwalfia Serpentia, a root

---

14. A Treatise on the Canon of Medicine of Avicenna incorporating a Translation of the First Book O. Cameron Gruner, M.D.(Lond) Published by Luzac & Co London. ISBN 13:2471678676916

that proved to be a potent and popular remedy for hypertension in the 1960s and well known to the Hakims for centuries before being exploited by the West. No doubt in this pharmacopoeia there are other drugs that need to be scientifically analyzed by random studies and double-blind clinical trials for their effectiveness.

The Contemporary Practice of Islamic Medicine

Although Islamic medicine continues to be practiced in many Muslim countries today, Western medicine has replaced the core of the health care system in most of them. The only countries where it has enjoyed a degree of official status are in the Indian subcontinent. In India, medical schools have been established where Tibb or Yūnānī medicine (translated as natural medicine or Greek medicine) continues to be taught. These schools give students instructed in Yūnānī concepts of medicine a formal diploma in Tibb or Yūnānī, which enables them to be licensed practitioners authorized to utilize this knowledge and therapeutics in their practice. Their certification, licensing, and supervision are controlled by the Indian Medical Council. In Pakistan, in the middle 1960s, the government under then-President Muhammad Ayyūb Khan ordered the official registration and licensing of traditional Hakīms (much to the chagrin of practitioners of modern medicine). Tibb also enjoys public popularity in other countries, including Afghanistan, Malaysia, and some countries in the Middle East, where there has recently been an increase in the number of practitioners.

Conclusion

The greatest challenge of Islamic medicine is not in its practice, therapeutics, or application, but in its adaptation to modern day needs. Thus, it is my belief that the fundamental challenge is not the way in which Islamic medicine is practiced, but the way in which it is defined. Somewhere in the late 16th and 17th centuries, a dichotomy developed between Islamic medicine and modern, or Western, medicine. This dichotomy was mainly related to the development of one civilization and the decline of another. Such cycles are an on-going fact of history. To say that one system of medicine is superior to another is perhaps akin to saying one antibiotic is superior to another based solely on chronology. Although one of them may have been discovered earlier, and one later, each continues to play its role in the treatment of a given ailment. The challenge is to study and define the interrelationship, and precisely define when one is more useful than another. By analog, the same might apply to these two different systems of medicine. The roles of each one needs to be defined. Each needs to be studied in the light of each other's progress, and mutually supplemented.

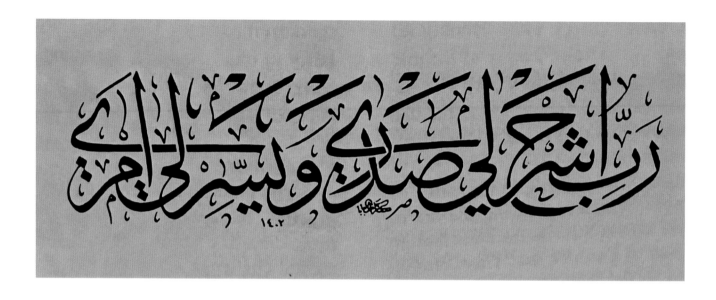

This article is from a talk presented by Dr. Nagamia at the 3rd. Annual Conference of the International Institute of Islamic Medicine (IIIM) held in Birmingham, United Kingdom from June 26-30, 1998. It was later modified and published in the Journal of Islamic Medicine:

JIMA: Volume 32, pages 111-120, 2000.It has been copy edited for inclusion in this current volume.

CHAPTER 3:

Contributors to the Islamic Civilization

Mahmood Hai, MD, FICS

a. A list of eminent contributors to the era (by century)

Century	Name	Country of Birth	Life Span (CE)
Seventh			
601–700	**Prophet Muhammad Bin Abdullah (PBUH)**	**Arabia**	**570–632 (610–632)**
	Rufaida al-Aslamia	**Arabia**	**Contemporary of the Prophet PBUH**
	Al-Shifa Bint Abdullah al-Adawiya	**Arabia**	**Contemporary of the Prophet PBUH**
	Ibn Atal (Ibn Uthal)		
	Al-Harit Ben-Kalada al-Taqafi		
	Ibn Abi Ramtha al-Tamimi		
	Masarjawaih		
	Nafi Ibn al-Harith		
	Abu Hafsa Yazid		
Eighth			
701–800			
	Abu Yahya Ibn al-Batriq	**Syria**	**730–815**
	Jabir Ibn Hayyan	**Iraq**	**Died 816**
	Jibril Ibn Bukhtishu	**Persia**	**781–828**
	Jafar al-Sadiq		
	Imam Ali Ibn Mousa al-Ridha		
Ninth			

801–900			
	Abu Yusuf Ibn Ishaq as Sabbah al-Kindi	**Iraq**	**801–873**
	Yuhanna Ibn Bukhtishu	**Persia**	**820–903**
	Hunayn Ibn Ishaq al-Ibadi	**Baghdad**	**826–901**
	Thabet Ibn Qurrah	**Turkey**	**826–901**
	Ali Ibn Sahl Rabban al-Tabari	**Persia**	**838–917**
	Abu Zayd Ahmed Ibn Sahl Balkhi	**Persia**	**850–934**
	Abu Bakr Ibn Zakariyya al-Razi (Rhazez)	**Persia**	**854–925**
	Ali Ibn Yusuf al-Jazari Ibn al-Jazzar (*The Viaticum*)	**Tunisia**	**895–979**
	Yahya Ibn Sarafyun		
	Yuhanna Ibn Masawaiyh		
	Shapur Ibn Sahl		
	Al-Bubather		
	Al-Ruhawi		
	Salmawaih Ibn Bunan		
	Yusuf al-Khuri		
Tenth			
901–1000			
	Abul Hasan al-Tabari	**Persia**	**916–986**
	Ali Ibn al-Abbas al-Majusi	**Persia**	**930–994**
	Muhammad Ibn Saad al-Tamimi	**Jerusalem**	**Died 990**
	Abul Qasim al-Zahrawi (Abulcasis)	**Spain**	**936–1013**
	Hasan Ibn al-Haytham	**Iraq**	**965–1040**
	Abdul Ali al-Husayn Ibn Sina (Avicenna)	**Persia**	**980–1037**
	Qusta Ibn Luqa		
	Abu ul-Ala Shirazi		
	Al-Natili		
	Qumri		
	Abu Zayd al-Balkhi		
	Isaac Israeli Ben Solomon		
	Al-Masihi		
	Muvaffak		
	Ibn Juljul		
	Al-Jabali		
	Al-Kashkari		
	Ibn Abi al-Ashath		
	Ibn al-Jazzar		

	Al-Kashkari		
	Ibrahim Ibn Baks		
	Abu al-Qasim Muqane'i		
	Abu Bakr Bokhari		
	Avon Ibn Aayon		
	Al-Biruni		
	Ali Ibn Ridwan		
	Abubakr al-Razi		
	Abu Sahl'Isa ibn Yahya al-Masihi		
	Abu Ula'l Shirazi		
	Eutychius of Alexandria		
	Mohammed Ibn Abdun al-Jabali		
Eleventh			
1001–1100			
	Abul-i-ala Ibn Zuhr (Avenzoar)	**Arabia**	**1094–1162**
	Ephraim Ibn al-Za'fran		
	Ibn al-Wafid		
	Ammar al-Mawsili		
	Abdollah Ibn Bukhtishu		
	Abu Ubayd al-Juziani		
	Al-Biruni		
	Ali Ibn Ridwan		
	Ibn Butlan		
	Al-Kirmani		
	Ibn al-Kattani		
	Ibn Jazla		
	Masawaih al-Mardini		
	Al-Ilaqi		
	Ibn al-Thahabi		
	Ibn Abi Sadiq		
	Ali Ibn Isa al-Kahhal		
	Ibn Hindu		
	Al-Badi al-Asturlabi		
	Avempace		
	Abu al-Bayan Ibn al-Mudawwar		
	Ahmad Ibn Farrokh		
	Zayn al-Din Gorgani		
	Serapion the Younger		

	Abu Alhakam'Al-Kirmani		
	Ali Ibn Yusuf al-Ilaqi		
	Jonah Ibn Janah		
Twelfth			
1101–1200			
	Muhadhdhab al-Din al-Baghdadi (Ibn Butlan)	**Iraq**	**1117–1213**
	Abdul Walid Ibn Rushd (Averroes)	**Spain**	**1126–1198**
	Ali Ibn Ahmad Ibn Hubal	**Iraq**	**1127–1213**
	Moses Ben Maimon (Maimonides)	**Spain**	**1135–1204**
	Abdallah Ibn Ahmad al-Malaqi (Ibn al-Baitar)	**Spain**	**1197–1248**
	Yaqub Ibn Ishaq al-Israili		
	Al-Turjali		
	Ibn Tufail		
	Al-Ghafiqi		
	Ibn Abi al-Hakam		
	Abul Barakat al-Baghdadi		
	Al-Samawal al-Maghribi		
	Ibn al-Tilmidh		
	Ibn Jumay		
	Abu Jafar Ibn Harun al-Turjali		
	Abu al-Bayan Ibn al-Mudawwar		
	Ahmad Ibn Farrokh		
	Zayn Aldin Gorgani		
	Avem Pace		
	Moshe Ben Maimon		
Thirteenth			
1201–1300			
	Al-al-Din Abu al-Hassan Ali Ibn al-Nafis	**Syria**	**1213–1288**
	Amin ud-Daula Farj Ibn al-Quff	**Syria**	**1232–1286**
	Ibn Tumlus		
	Sa'ad al-Dawla		
	Al-Sharazuri		
	Rashidun al-Suri		
	As-Suwaydi		
	Amin al-Din Rashid al-Din Vatvat		
	Abraham Ben Moses Ben Maimon		
	Daud Abu al-Fadl		
	Al-Dakhwar Ibn al-Usaibia		

	Joseph Ben Judah of Ceuta		
	Ibn al-Raqqam		
	Abd al-Latif al-Baghdadi		
	Zakaraiya al-Qazwini		
	Najib ad-Din-e-Samarqandi		
	Qutub al-Din al-Shirazi		
	Hussam al-din al-Jarrahi		
Fourteenth			
1301–1400			
	Mansur Ibn Yusuf Ibn Ilyas	**Persia**	**1380–1422**
	Sabuncuoglu Serafeddin	**Turkey**	**1385–1468**
	Ibn al-Akfani		
	Muhammad Ibn Mahmud Amuli		
	Al-Nagawri		
	Aqsara'i		
	Zayn-e-Attar		
	Jagmini		
	Mas'ud Ibn Muhammad Sijzi		
	Najm al-Din al-Shirazi		
	Nakhshabi		
	Sadid al-Din al-Kazaruni		
	Yusuf Ibn Ismail al-Kutubi		
	Ibn Shuayb		
	Ibn al-Khatib		
	Rashid al-Din Hamdani		
Fifteenth			
1401–1500			
	Abu Sa'id al-Afif		
	Muhammad Ali Astrabadi		
	Husayni Isfahani		
	Burhan-ud-Din Kermani		
	Al-Harawi		
	Nurbakhshi		
	Shaykh Muhammad Ibn Thaleb		
Sixteenth			
1501–1600			
	Dawud Ibn Umar al-Antaki	**Syria**	**1543–1599**
	Hakim-e-Gilani		

	Abul Qasim Ibn Mohammed al-Ghassani		
	Taqi ad-Din Muhammad Ibn Ma'ruf		
	Sultan Ali Khorasani		
Seventeenth			
1601–1700			
	Abd el-Razzaq al-Jazairi		

b. Thirty-One Eminent Contributors to the Field of Medicine

1. Prophet Muhammad Bin Abdullah (PBUH)
2. Rufaida al-Aslamia
3. Al-Shifa Bint Abdullah al-Adawiya (Layla)
4. Abu Yahya Ibn al-Batriq
5. Jabir Ibn Hayyan
6. Jibril Ibn Bukhtishu and the Bukhtishu family
7. Abu Yusuf Ibn Ishaq as-Sabbah al-Kindi
8. Yuhanna Ibn Bukhtishu
9. Hunayn Ibn Ishaq al-Ibadi
10. Thabet Ibn Qurrah
11. Ali Ibn Sahl Rabban al-Tabari
12. Abu Zayd Ahmed Ibn Sahl Balkhi
13. Abu Bakr Ibn Zakariyya al-Razi (Rhazez)
14. Ali Ibn Yusuf al-Jazari Ibn al-Jazzar (*The Viaticum*)
15. Abul Hasan al-Tabari
16. Ali Ibn al-Abbas al-Majusi (Hally Abbas)
17. Muhammad Ibn Saad al-Tamimi
18. Abul Qasim al-Zahrawi (Abulcasis)
19. Hasan Ibn al-Haytham
20. Ibn Sina (Avicenna)
21. Abul-i-ala Ibn Zuhr (Avenzoar)
22. Muhadhdhab al-Din al-Baghdadi (Ibn Butlan)
23. Abdul Walid Ibn Rushd (Averroes)
24. Ali Ibn Ahmad Ibn Hubal
25. Moses Ben Maimon (Maimonides)
26. Abdallah Ibn Ahmad al-Malaqi (Ibn al-Baitar)
27. Al-al-Din abu al-Hassan Ali Ibn al-Nafis
28. Amin ud-Daula Farj Ibn al-Quff
29. Mansur Ibn Yusuf Ibn Ilyas
30. Sabuncuoglu Serafeddin
31. Dawud Ibn Umar al-Antaki

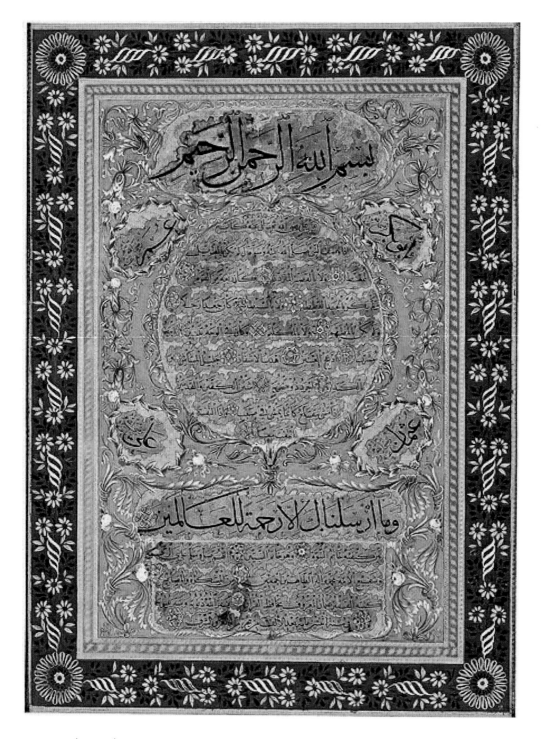

Hilye (Hilya) – Ottoman calligraphy panel; the text describes the physical appearance of the Prophet Muhammad (PBUH) by Hafiz Osman 17th Century

c. Short Biographies of the Contributors to Medicine

1. Prophet Muhammad Bin Abdullah (PBUH)

Tibb-e-Nabawi is the divine gift of the complete code of medicine that God revealed to the Prophet Muhammad (PBUH), resulting in the following sayings of the Prophet:

"Every illness has a cure, and when proper cure is applied to the disease, it heals by God's will."

"God has not sent down a disease except that He has also sent down its cure."

The Prophet used medicine for himself and his family and is said to have advised, "When illness happens, seek medicine." He also mentioned the use of foods, herbs, and *hijamah* (cupping). The Prophet promoted healthy, clean living and prevention of diseases. It is mentioned in as-Sayuti's sixteenth-century manuscript on al-Tibb al-Nawabi that the Prophet not only instructed sick people to take medicine, but he himself invited expert physicians for this purpose. In his famous book *Muqaddimah*, Ibn Khaldun quotes the Prophet (PBUH): "The stomach is the house of illness, and abstinence (from food) is the important medicine." The most famous physician at the time of the Prophet (PBUH) was al-Harith Bin Kalada al-Taqafi, who lived in Gondishapur.

Please refer to Chapter 6: "The Islamic Principles of Hygiene as Practiced by Muhammad Bin Abdullah [PBUH]."

Folio from al-Tibb al-Nawabi created in the era of Suleiman the Magnificient

2. Rufaida al-Aslamia

Please refer to Chapter 9: "Muslim Female Physicians and Healthcare Providers in Islamic History."

3. Al-Shifa Bint Abdullah al-Adawiya (Layla)

Please refer to Chapter 9: "Muslim Female Physicians and Healthcare Providers in Islamic History."

4. Abu Yahya Ibn al-Batriq (730–815 CE)

Al-Batriq was a Syrian scholar who pioneered the translation of ancient Greek texts into Arabic, a major early figure in the transmission of the classics. He translated for Caliph al-Mansur the major medical works of Galen and Hippocrates and compiled the encyclopedia *Kitab Sirr al-Asrar*, a book of the science of government that was translated into Latin in the twelfth century as *Secretum Secretorum* (*Secret of Secrets*). Besides medicine it dealt with statecraft, ethics, physiognomy, astrology, alchemy, and magic.

5. Jabir Ibn Hayyan (721–815 CE)

Ibn Hayyan, was born in Tous (Iran) and died in Kufa (Iraq). A Muslim alchemist, he was known as the father of Arabic chemistry, which in turn formed the basis of modern chemistry. Ibn Hayyan liberated chemistry from superstition and transformed it into a science. He perfected the process of purification and crystallization. He discovered and extracted citric acid from lemons and acetic acid from vinegar, which was later used in the pharmaceutical industry. He also authored hundreds of books, including *Kitab al-Kimia (The Book of Alchemy)*. In his later years, he fell into disrepute with the caliph and was placed under house arrest. He died at the age of ninety-four.

6. Jibril Ibn Bukhtishu and the Bukhtishu Family

In 762, when Baghdad became the center of the Abbasid caliphate, Caliph al-Mansur invited the head physician of the Gondishapur school, Jirjis Bukhtishu I, to treat his illness. Jirjis was a Nestorian Christian whose name meant "Jesus has saved." Jirjis returned to his hometown before his death but left his son, Jibril Bukhtishu II, who established his practice in Baghdad and became a prominent physician. Because of their elite relationship with the caliphate, the family continued to produce physicians for eight generations, from the eighth century to the eleventh. Many of them, including Juris Bukhtishu II, Yuhanna Ibn Bukhtishu, Ubaidullah Ibn Bukhtishu, and Jibril Bukhtishu III, made major contributions to Islam's golden age.

7. Abu Yusuf Ibn Ishaq as-Sabbah al-Kindi (801–873 CE)

Al-Kindi, who was born in Kufa and died in Baghdad, was an Arab Muslim philosopher, mathematician, physician, and music theorist who is hailed as the father of Arab philosophy. A polymath, he wrote hundreds of original treatises on subjects ranging from metaphysics, ethics, logic, and psychology to medicine, pharmacology, mathematics, astronomy, astrology, and optics. In the practical field, he dealt with topics like perfumes, swords, jewels, glass, dyes, zoology, tides, mirrors, meteorology, and earthquakes. He introduced Indian numerals to the Islamic world and subsequently relabeled them as Arabic numerals.

Using his mathematical and medical expertise, he was able to develop a scale that allowed doctors to quantify the potency of their medications. In his study of Muslim theology, he believed revelation was a superior source of knowledge to reason because it incorporated matters of faith that reason could not uncover. Under the militant orthodoxy of Caliph al-Mutawakkil, he was persecuted and beaten and died as a lonely man during the reign of Caliph al-Mu'tamid.

8. Yuhanna Ibn Bukhtishu

Yuhanna Ibn Bukhtishu was known to be the illegitimate son of Jibril Ibn Bukhtishu referring to item 6 in the list mentioned in the previous section. The name is composed of the Persian word *Bukht*, meaning saved, and the Syriac word *Ishu*, meaning Jesus. He wrote several treatises on the astrological knowledge necessary for a physician; a copy is saved at the National Library of Medicine. Yuhanna served as the physician to the caliphs al-Wathiq and al-Mutawakkil in Baghdad.

9. Hunayn Ibn Ishaq al-Ibadi (CE 809–873)

Ibn Ishaq was born in al-Hirah (Iraq) and died in Baghdad. He was an influential Arab Nestorian Christian physician, scientist, and scholar. He studied Greek and became known among the Arabs as the sheikh of the translators. His translations from Greek science laid the foundation for Islamic medicine. In his lifetime, Ibn Ishaq translated 116 works and produced 36 of his own books, 21 of which addressed the field of medicine. The Abbasid caliph, al-Mamun, recognized Ibn Ishaq's talents and placed him in charge of the House of Wisdom in Baghdad. His chief medical contribution was in ophthalmology through his innovative *Book of the Ten Treaties of the Eye*. Caliph al-Mutawakkil tested Ibn Ishaq by asking him to formulate a poison. He refused to do so, explaining the physician's oath that required him to help and not harm his patients.

10. Thabet Ibn Qurrah (CE 836–901)

Thabet was born in Upper Mesopotamia, during the Abbasid era, and died in Baghdad. He was an Arab physician, mathematician, astronomer, and translator in the second half of the ninth century. He originally belonged to an astronomical group called the Sabians. He worked as a money changer before he came to Baghdad. His first language was Syriac, but he was fluent in Greek and Arabic, which served him well when translating classical texts. He translated the works of Archimedes, Euclid, and Ptolemy and founded a school of translation in Baghdad. Although his major works were in the fields of astronomy, physics, and mathematics, he also made contributions to the science of medicine. His major contribution was translating summaries of the works of Hippocrates and Galen. In the field of mechanics, he was the founder of statics. He calculated the length of a solar year, being off by only two seconds. Later in life he became a friend and courtier of Caliph al-Mu'tadid. His son Sinan Ibn Thabit became a renowned physician and director of a hospital in Baghdad.

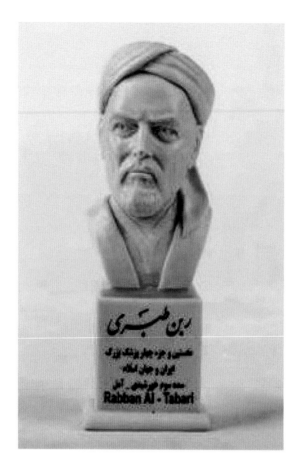

Statue of Ali Ibn Sahl Rabban al-Tabari

II. Ali Ibn Sahl Rabban al-Tabari (778–864 CE)

Al-Tabari, born in Amol (Iran), was a Persian Muslim scholar, physician, and psychologist who produced the first encyclopedia of medicine, titled *Firdous al-Hikmah* (*Paradise of Wisdom*). It is divided into seven sections and thirty parts, with 360 chapters in total covering every aspect of medicine known at that time. He spoke Syriac and Greek fluently and transcribed books of antiquity in meticulous calligraphic Arabic. His most famous student was Muhammad Ibn Zakariya al-Razi, who overshadowed his fame.

Al-Tabari came from a very educated and respected Christian family in Iran. His name derives from a mountainous region located on the Caspian coast of northern Iran. He converted to Islam at a very late age. He received his education in the medical field but was also tutored by his father in natural sciences, mathematics, philosophy, literature, and calligraphy. He left twelve books, most of which are concerned with medicine. He was the first to discover that pulmonary tuberculosis was a contagious disease.

Outside the field of science, Al-Tabari was involved in interreligious discussions and authored two critical works on religion. He was known as a man of wisdom with intellectual and administrative abilities. The Abbasid caliph, al-Mu'tasim, summoned him to Baghdad where later he served as private physician to the new caliph, al-Mutawakkil and became his close companion. Al-Tabari passed away at the age of seventy-six in Baghdad.

12. Abu Zayd Ahmed Ibn Sahl Balkhi (850–934 CE)

Al-Balkhi was a Persian Muslim polymath, geographer, mathematician, physician, psychologist, and scientist born in Balkh, Persia. He was a disciple of al-Kindi and is believed to be the first to understand that mental illness can have both psychological and physiological causes. He classified emotional disorders into four types: 1. Fear and anxiety 2. Anger and aggression 3. Sadness and depression. 4. Obsessions.

On a personal level, Al-Balkhi had a reserved and isolated character. His face was covered with scars from a bout of smallpox. In his early years he traveled to Baghdad and spent a decade with al-Kindi studying philosophy, astronomy, natural sciences, and disciplines of the Quran. On his return to Balkh, the ruler of Balkh gave him an appointment as a writer for which he was handsomely rewarded.

Of the many books ascribed to him, his famous work *Masalih al-Abdan wa al-Anfus* (*Sustenance of Body and Soul*) is considered foundational to modern psychology and psychiatry. Al-Balkhi developed his ideas on mental health from the verses of the Quran and the hadiths of the Prophet Mohammed (PBUH). The first to successfully describe diseases related to both the soul (*al-Tibb al-Ruhani*) and the body (*Tibb al-Qalb*), he argued that "since man's construction is from both his soul and his body, therefore, human existence cannot be healthy without the *ishtibak* (interweaving) of soul and body." He further argued that "if the body gets sick, the *nafs* (psyche) loses much of its cognitive and comprehensive ability and fails to enjoy the desirous aspects of life," and that "if the *nafs* falls ill, the body may also find no joy in life and may eventually develop a physical illness." This is what in modern medicine we refer to as psychosomatic illnesses. Al-Balkhi was also the first to differentiate between neurosis and psychosis, which led to his understanding of medical psycho-physiology, cognitive therapy, and psychosomatic medicine. Although sexuality was not much discussed in his day, al-Balkhi explored the subject in detail, mentioning in his work that the act of remaining abstinent is "unnatural" and could lead to physical ailments. He passed away at the age of eighty-four in Balkh, leaving a rich heritage of knowledge.

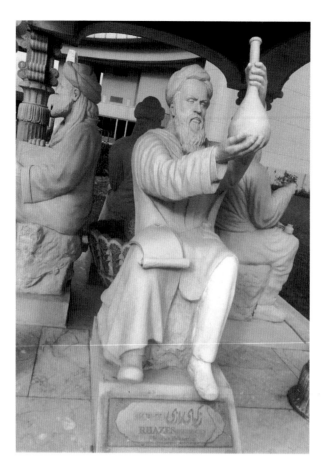

Al-Razi's marble statue at the United Nation's office in Vienna

13. Abu Bakr Ibn Zakariyya al-Razi (Rhazez) (864–935 CE)

Al-Razi's full name was Abu Bakr Muhammad Ibn Zakariyya, and he was given the title of Fakhr al-Din al-Razi. His Latinized name was Rhazes. Al-Razi, who was born and died in Rayy, Iran, was a Persian physician, philosopher, and alchemist widely considered one of the most important figures in the history of medicine. He studied music and became a skillful flutist.

Al-Razi was also known as a comprehensive, logical thinker who made fundamental and enduring contributions to various fields of medicine, logic, astronomy, and grammar. He is particularly remembered for numerous advances in medicine based on his observations and discovery. An early proponent of experimental medicine, he became a successful doctor. He first became the court physician of Prince Abu Saleh Al-Mansur, the ruler of Khorosan, and later the chief physician of Baghdad Hospital.

As a teacher of medicine, al-Razi attracted students of all backgrounds and interests and was said to be compassionate and devoted to the service of his patients, whether rich or poor. As a person, al-Razi was known to be generous and charitable to the poor, treating them without payment. In his later years he even wrote a treatise "Man La Yahdruhu al-Tabib," offering medical advice to anyone "Who Has No Physician to Attend Him." He was the first to distinguish clinically between smallpox and measles.

Al-Razi published several books and wrote over 200 manuscripts on a variety of subjects, including religion. Certain of these were recognized by medieval European practitioners and profoundly influenced medical education in the west. Several of his books were translated into Latin, French, Italian, Hebrew, and Greek. Some volumes of his work *Al-Mansuri*, namely "On Surgery" and "A General Book on Therapy," became part of the medical curriculum in European universities. Additionally, he has been described as the father of pediatrics and a pioneer of obstetrics and ophthalmology. The pupillary response to light was one of his discoveries.

Al-Razi defined medicine as "the art concerned with preserving healthy bodies, in combating disease, and in restoring health to the sick." His contributions to medicine include works on medical ethics, psychology, psychotherapy, meningitis, and pharmacy, and many monumental books on medicine and alchemy. His book *Al-Murshid* emphasized seven important principles for the preservation of health. Another of his famous books was called *Al-Hawi* (*The Complete Text*). It consisted of twenty-two volumes and became the primary medical textbook in many medical schools in Europe.

Al-Razi spent the last few years of his life in his hometown of Rayy suffering with glaucoma and cataracts, which led to total blindness. One of his former students from Tabaristan came to look after him. Al-Razi rewarded him for his intentions but sent him back home, aware that his final days were drawing near. Al-Biruni, who considered al-Razi his mentor, was one of the first to write his biography and included a bibliography of his numerous works. After his death, al-Razi's fame spread beyond the Middle East to medieval Europe. The library at Peterborough Abbey contains a catalog of ten books on medicine authored by al-Razi.

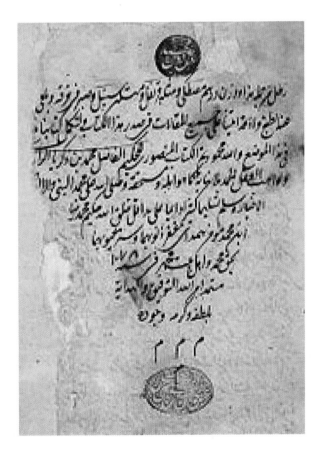

Colophon of al-Razi's Book of Medicine for Mansur

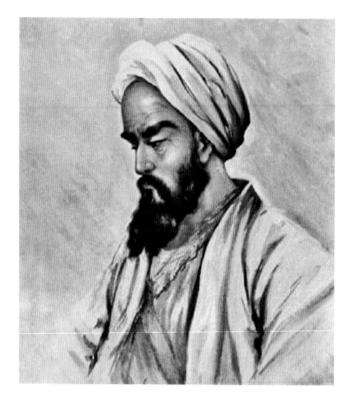

A colored portrait of al-Razi

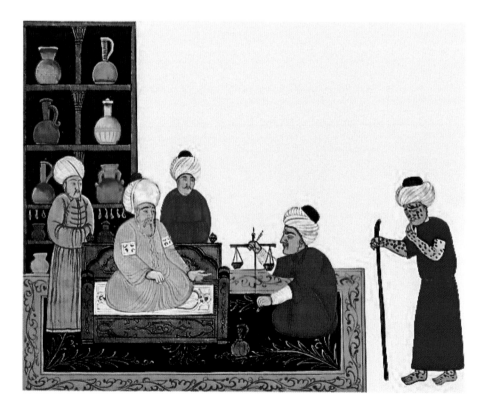

A patient with smallpox arriving at al-Razi's clinic

THE CONTRIBUTIONS OF ISLAMIC CIVILIZATION TO MEDICINE

14. Ali Ibn Yusuf al-Jazari Ibn al-Jazzar, author of *The Viaticum*, 898–980 CE

Born and buried in Kairouan, Tunisia, al-Jazzar was a Muslim Arab physician famous for his writings on Islamic medicine. He learned the Quran in his youth and pursued his study of grammar, Islamic law (*fiqh*), and history. His father and uncle were physicians. They taught him medicine. Later he came under the tutelage of Isaac Ben Salomon, a local Jewish physician. Al-Jazzar was calm and quiet and avoided festivities. After a busy day of medical consultation, he taught students at his home. Al-Jazzar possessed a rich library that covered medicine and other disciplines. The Emir of Kairouan, who valued his friendship and medical skills, prevented him from going to Cordoba, the era's most famous seat of learning.

Al-Jazzar charged fees for his medical services, pharmaceutical preparations, and for house calls. By the time of his death, he had earned over 100,000 grams worth of gold dinars. He identified contagious diseases a millennium ago. He was the first physician to diagnose leprosy, explaining the disease in scientific terms and recommending measures to contain it, although the Norwegian Gerhard Hansen is popularly regarded as the first physician to identify the main cause of leprosy in 1873.

Al-Jazzar composed several books on grammar, history, jurisprudence, and medicine. The most important of these was *Zad al-Musafir* (*The Viaticum*), a handbook of medicine designed for clinical teaching that covered all organs from head to toe. Each disease was listed with its known symptoms, suggested treatment, and sometimes even the prognosis. It was translated into Latin, Greek, and Hebrew and then copied and recopied and printed in France and Italy in the sixteenth century. *The Viaticum* was not only used to teach in medical schools but was also a handy source for busy practitioners.

Al-Jazzar's other books were *Kitab Tibb al-Mashayikh*, which dealt with geriatric medicine; *Risala fi Asbab al-Wafah*, a treatise on causes of death; and other books on sleep disorders, forgetfulness, pediatrics, sexual disorders, and medicine for the poor. Al-Jazzar died at the age of eighty-four.

15. Abul Hasan al-Tabari (916–986 CE)

Abul Hasan, who was born in Tabaristan and died in Tarunja, Iran, was a tenth-century Persian physician. In his youth he served the Abbasid caliph, al-Baridi, together with his teacher, Abu Mahir Shirazi. Later he was appointed the physician of Rukn al-Dawla, a ruler of the Buyid dynasty. Although he wrote many valuable articles on different medical sciences, he is most famous for authoring the ten volumes of the *Kitab al-Mu'alaja al-Buqratiya* (*Hippocratic Treatments*), an important Arabic-language medical encyclopedia based on the works of Hippocrates that was used as a reference for many centuries. Abul Hasan was known as a creative and innovative physician who avoided emulating treatments without investigating and examining them. He paid adequate attention to philosophy and medical ethics, citing other scholars' works, seeing the need for clinical and hospital training, and emphasizing indigenous therapy and responsible treatment. He is credited with the discovery of Scabies (*Sarcoptes scabe)i*. He also addressed the treatment of migraine headaches.

16. Ali Ibn al-Abbas al-Majusi (Hally Abbas) (930–994 CE)

Al-Majusi, born in Ahvaz, Iran, and died in Shiraz, Iran, was a Persian physician and psychologist who is considered the pioneer of psychophysiology and psychosomatic medicine. His ancestors were Zoroastrian, but he himself was a Muslim. Al-Majusi is best known for his *Kitab Kamil as-Sina'a at-Tibbiya* (*Complete Book of the Medical Art*), a work completed in 980 CE and was dedicated to Emir Adud al-Daula Fana Khusraw of the Buyid dynasty. The book is a more systematic and concise encyclopedia than al-Razi's *Al-Hawi* and Ibn Sina's *Canon of Medicine*. It was later named *Kitab al-Malakiyy* (*Royal Book*). The book is divided into twenty discourses, the first ten of which deal with theory and the second ten with the practice of medicine. In 1087 CE it was translated into Latin and used as a textbook in the medical school in Salerno, Italy. More complete and much better translations followed in 1492 and 1523 when it was used all over Europe as *Hally Abbas's Textbook of Medicine*. It also established the basic concepts of dietetics, the human capillary system, and pregnancy. Al-Majusi's work emphasized the need for a healthy relationship between doctors and patients and his medical ethics laid the foundation of a scientific methodology very similar to modern biomedical research.

He also described the neuroanatomy, neurobiology, and neurophysiology of the brain. Various mental disorders were first recognized by him, including sleeping sickness, memory loss, hypochondriasis, coma, meningitis, vertigo, epilepsy, love sickness, and hemiplegia. He found a correlation between physical and mental health and concluded that "joy and contentment can bring a better living status to many who would otherwise be sick and miserable due to unnecessary sadness, fear, worry and anxiety." Al-Majusi's book discusses diet, exercise, and even bathing as beneficial for health.

In dealing with medicines, al-Majusi states the best way to determine the effects of a drug is to test it on healthy people as well as the sick and to keep careful records of the results. In his book he described a classification system of drugs based on their properties and detailed methods of preparing pills, syrups, powders, and ointments. One treatment al-Majusi discusses is the treatment of aneurysm, a bulge resulting from weakness of an arterial wall. For smaller arteries, he advised physicians to cut open the patient's flesh to expose the blood vessel and then to tie it off at either end of the aneurysm with silk thread. This technique is still used today. For larger blood vessels, he advised not to tie them off as it would lead to death from blood loss and circulation. As a physician he believed in using diet and psychotherapy as the first step toward healing, failing which he recommended pharmaceuticals and surgery.

The emir, al-Daula, was a great patron of medicine and founded a hospital in Shiraz, Persia, in 981 CE. Later, al-Adudi Hospital was established in Baghdad and al-Majusi was made the physician in charge.

17. Muhammad Ibn Saad al-Tamimi (909–990 CE)

Al-Tamimi, who was born in Jerusalem and died in Egypt, was an Arab physician and highly regarded alchemist. He spent his early years in and around Jerusalem, where he studied medicine under the tutelage of al-Hasan Ibn Abi Nu'yam and a Christian monk, Abna Zecharia Ben Thawabah. Al-Tamimi possessed an uncommon knowledge of plants and their properties. Because of his highly coveted abilities, he served as the personal physician to the governor of Ramla, al-Hasan Bin Abdullah Bin Tughj al-Mastouli. In 970 he was invited to Cairo to render his services in Egypt. He prospered in his medical practice and wrote a medical work for the vizier, Yaqub Ibn Killis, under the Fatimid caliphate. Al-Tamimi specialized in compounding simple drugs and medicines and is especially known for the antidote he developed for snakebite and other poisons. It had exceptional qualities and was named *tiryaq al-faruq*, the antidote of salvation. His most prized medical work is *The Guidebook to Basics in Food and Nutrition and the Properties of Non-compounded Medicines*, known under the abbreviated name *Al-Murshid*.

Only portions of al-Tamimi's seminal work have survived. Sections of his original work were copied in 1270 CE and are preserved at the US National Library of Medicine. His work on *materia medica* is an invaluable source for understanding the curative remedies in use during the early Muslim era in Syria and Jerusalem.

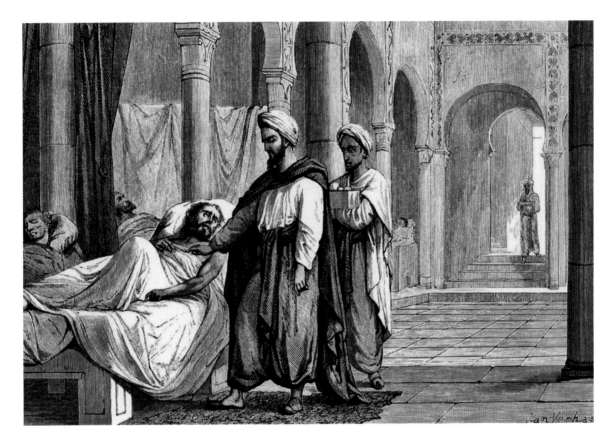

Al-Zahrawi (Abulcasis) attending to a patient in the hospital in Cordoba

18. Abul Qasim al-Zahrawi (Abulcasis) (936–1013 CE)

Al-Zahrawi, who was born in Madinat al-Zahra, Spain and died in Cordoba, was an Arab Andalusian physician, surgeon, and chemist. He is considered the greatest surgeon of the Middle Ages and has been referred to as the father of modern surgery. Al-Zahrawi's pioneering contributions to the field of surgical procedures and instruments had an enormous impact in the East and West well into the modern period. Some of his discoveries are applied in medical practice to this day. He pioneered the use of catgut and many of his surgical instruments are still used with some modifications. He was the first physician to identify the hereditary nature of hemophilia and described abdominal pregnancy as a subtype of ectopic pregnancy. The root cause of paralysis was another of his discoveries. He developed surgical instruments specifically for caesarean sections and for cataract eye surgeries.

Al-Zahrawi lived most of his life in Cordoba, where he studied, taught, and practiced medicine and surgery. Many of the details of his life and work were destroyed two years before his death when the caliphate succumbed to civil war.

Al-Zahrawi was a court physician to the Andalusian caliph, al-Hakam II, and devoted his entire life to the advancement of medicine as a whole and surgery in particular. He specialized in curing diseases by cauterization, for which he invented several new devices, establishing the basis for cautery as used in modern surgery. He was the first to treat warts. He invented several devices used during surgery for inspecting the interior of the urethra, throat, ear, and other organs.

Al-Zahrawi's principal work is *Kitab al-Tasrif*, a thirty-volume encyclopedia of medical practices completed in 1000 CE. He stressed the importance of learning the basic sciences.

"Before practicing one should be familiar with the science of anatomy and the function of organs so that he will understand them, recognize their shape, understand their connections and know their borders. Also, he should know the bones, nerves and muscles, their numbers, their origin and insertions, the arteries and veins, their start and end. These anatomical and physiological bases are important and as Hippocrates said, "Many doctors have the title, but real physicians are very few." If one does not comprehend anatomy and physiology, he may commit a mistake that can kill the patient".

In *Kitab al-Tasrif*, al-Zahrawi covered a broad range of topics, including surgery, medicine, orthopedics, ophthalmology, urology, pharmacology, nutrition, dentistry, childbirth, and pathology. The first volume deals with the general principles of medicine; the second addresses pathology while most of the other volumes focus on pharmacology and drugs. The last volume is the most celebrated and deals with surgery. Al-Zahrawi stated that he chose to discuss surgery in the last volume because he considered surgery the highest form of medicine. He emphasized that a doctor must not practice surgery until he becomes well versed in the other branches of medicine. He took pains to describe each procedure in detail, including the ligature of arteries and stripping of varicose veins, which is still practiced in the same manner today. In one section of his book is a detailed description of the types of skull fractures, how to diagnose them, and how to surgically treat them. He used wax and alcohol to stop bleeding from the skull during cranial surgery. He developed non-penetrating trephines to open the skull without damaging the soft tissue beneath it.

Al-Zahrawi was the first to teach the lithotomy position for vaginal surgeries and described the tracheostomy operation he had to perform as an emergency on one of his servants. He also described in detail the procedure for ligating the temporal artery for the treatment of persistent migraine, a procedure that is enjoying a revival in the twenty-first century.

Al-Zahrawi also became an eminent surgeon and was appointed as the court physician of the renowned Caliph of Cordoba, Abdel Rahman III. He spent a productive life practicing medicine and surgery, continuing his medical writings. He died at the age of eighty-three.

(See picture of instruments invented by al-Zahrawi)

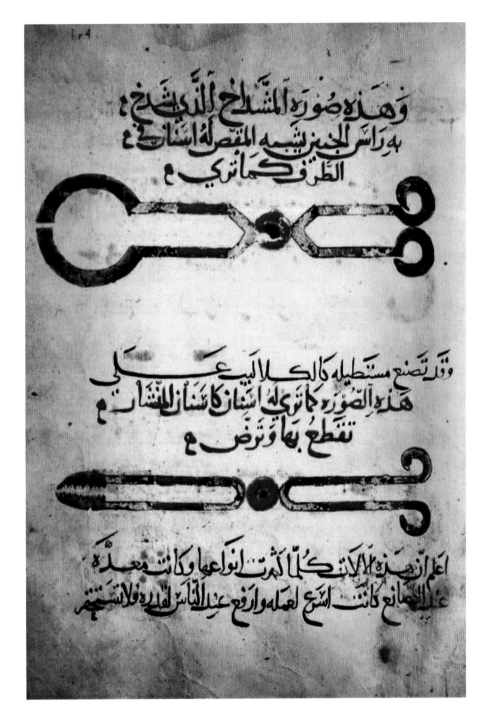

Folio showing surgical forceps developed and used by al-Zahrawi (Abulcasis)

19. Hasan Ibn al-Haytham (965–1040 CE)

Hasan Ibn al-Haytham, who was born in Basra, Iraq, and died in Cairo, was an Arab mathematician, astronomer, physicist, and physician who is referred to as the father of modern optics. He made significant contributions to the principles of optics and understanding of visual perception, which paved the way for the modern science of physical optics. Ibn al-Haytham was an early proponent of the argument that a hypothesis must be supported by experiments based on confirmable procedures or mathematical evidence. His pioneering concept of scientific methodology 500 years before the Renaissance, establishes him as among the first true scientists. Ibn al-Haytham was the first to explain that vision occurs when light reflects from an object and then passes to the eyes and is perceived in the brain.

Ibn al-Haytham's initial influences were in the study of religion and service to humanity, but his views came into conflict with the society of that time. As a result, he chose to delve into the study of mathematics and science. Later he was given the position of the vizier in Basra. Based on his brilliant reputation he was invited to Cairo by the Fatimid caliph, al-Hakim bi-Amr Allah, to regulate the flooding of the Nile. His project became impractical and failed, raising the ire of the caliph, and leading to house arrest and confiscation of his possessions. During this time, he wrote his influential *Book of Optics* (*Kitab al-Manazir*), and after the death of the caliph, he was given freedom. He continued to live in Cairo in the neighborhood of the famous al-Azhar University. He lived on the proceeds of his literary production until his death in 1040. A book written in Ibn al-Haytham's own handwriting is preserved in the Aya Sofía Museum in Istanbul, Turkey.

The *Book of Optics*, Ibn al-Haytham's most famous treatise, was written in seven volumes between 1011 CE and 1020 CE. By combining Galen's knowledge of the anatomy and physiology of the eye Ptolemy's optics from Ptolemy, and Euclid's mathematical studies of light rays, he explained the formation of a coherent image. He studied the process of sight, the structure of the eye, image formation in the eye, and the visual system. Many modern scholars agree that al-Haytham should be credited with a significant number of discoveries and theories that have been wrongly attributed to Western Europeans writing centuries later. His thoughts on vision and theory of light survived through the Middle Ages and inspired much activity in optics from the thirteenth century to the seventeenth. His book was translated into Latin by the end of the twelfth century and into Italian and other European languages at the end of the fourteenth century.

Ibn al-Haytham has been called the father of photography based on his work on the *camera obscura*, in which he explained the inversion of an image when it passes through a pinhole. While investigating a partial solar eclipse, he made the following statement: "The image of the sun at the time of the eclipse, unless it is total, demonstrates that when its light passes through a narrow round hole and is cast on a plane opposite to the hole, it takes on the form of a sickle moon". To explain the phenomenon of refraction, he described several experimental observations using mechanical analogies.

Ibn al-Haytham also set a standard for scientific methodology. He clearly stated, "The duty of the man who investigates the writings of scientists, if learning the truth is his goal, is to make himself an enemy of all that he reads, and … attack it from every side. He should also suspect himself as he performs his critical examination of it, so that he may avoid falling into either prejudice or leniency."

Al-Haytham was a true polymath whose works and contributions spread far into astronomy, geometry, calculus, engineering, philosophy, and theology. Regarding the relation of objective truth and God, he made this statement: "I constantly sought knowledge and truth, and it became my belief that for gaining access to the effulgence and closeness to God, there is no better way than that of searching for truth and knowledge."

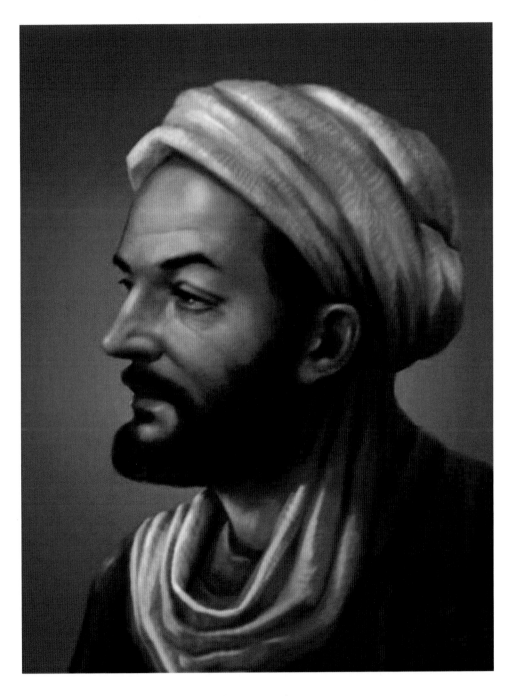

Potrait of Ibn Sina (Avicenna) as a young physician

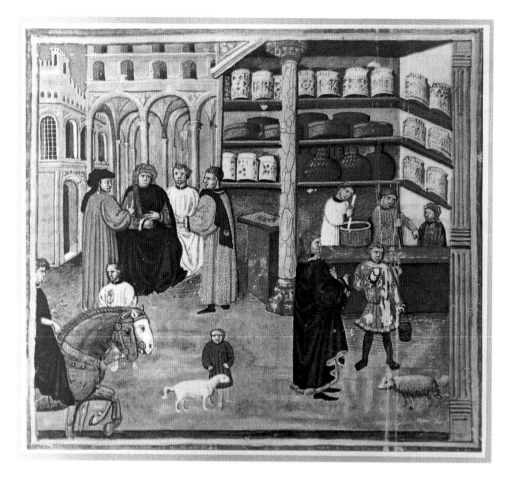

Ibn Sina (Avicenna) expounding pharmacy to his pupils

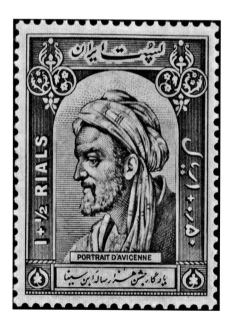

Stamp printed in Iran to honor Ibn Sina (Avicenna)

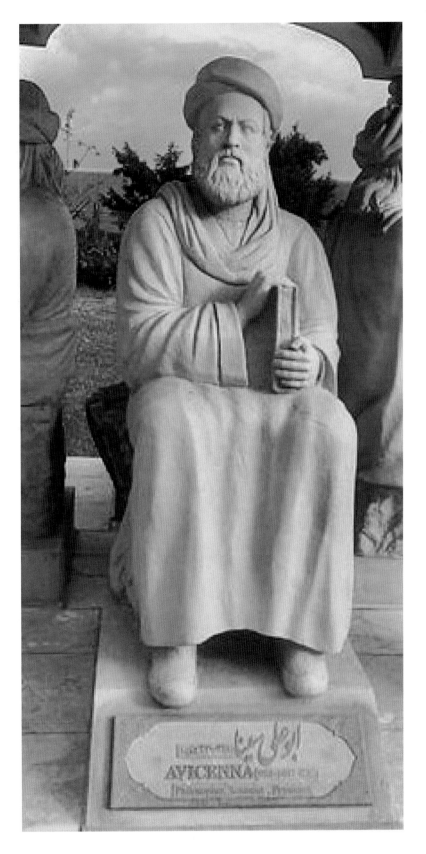

Statue of Ibn Sina (Avicenna) at the United Nations office in Vienna

Well-preserved copy of *al-Qanun fi al-Tibb* (The Canon of Medicine)
by Ibn Sina (Avicenna) published in 1025 AD

20. Ibn Sina (Avicenna) (980–1037 CE)

Ibn Sina, was born in Afshona, Uzbekistan and died in Hamadan, Iran. This Persian polymath is regarded as one of the most significant physicians, astronomers, philosophers, and writers of the golden age of Islamic civilization as well as the father of modern medicine. Of the 450 works he is believed to have written around 240 have survived, including 150 works on philosophy and 40 on medicine. His most famous works are *The Book of Healing*, a philosophical and scientific encyclopedia, and *The Canon of Medicine*, a purely medical encyclopedia. The *Canon* became a standard medical text at many universities and remained in use as late as 1650. Besides medicine and philosophy, Ibn Sina's writings cover astronomy, alchemy, geography, geology, psychology, Islamic theology, logic, mathematics, physics, and works of poetry.

His father, Abd-Allah, was a native of Balkh but served as the governor of a village close to Bukhara. A few years later the family settled in Bukhara, a center of learning that attracted many scholars. Although his father and brother had converted to Ismailism, a Shia subset of Islam, Ibn Sina remained an adherent of the Sunni Hanafi school. He was first schooled in the Quran and literature and by the age of ten had become a *hafiz*, memorizing the whole scripture. On the side, he learned arithmetic from an Indian grocer and Hanafi jurisprudence from a jurist, Ismail al-Zahid. Seeing the bright potential of his son, Ibn Sina's father invited a famous physician and philosopher, Abdallah al-Natili, to live in their house and educate Ibn Sina. Receiving further tutoring by well-known physicians Abu Mansur Qumri and Abu Sahl al-Masihi, Ibn Sina became a physician at the age of seventeen. When he turned twenty-one his father passed away. Ibn Sina was made governor of his village, and a few years later he entered the service of the Ma'munid ruler of the region, Abu al-Hasan Ali.

Ibn Sina established centers of learning wherever he went. In 1014 CE he was appointed court physician by the Buyid ruler Majd al-Dawla. During this phase he completed *The Canon of Medicine* and started writing the *Book of Healing*. Ibn Sina's life was extremely strenuous at this time. All day he was busy with his role as vizier and a great part of his night was spent lecturing and writing.

Ibn Sina wrote extensively on Islamic philosophy, especially the subjects of logic, ethics, and metaphysics, and was influenced by earlier philosophers like al-Farabi. He made an argument for the existence of God that would become known as the "Proof of the Truthful". Present-day historians of philosophy call this one of the most influential medieval arguments for God's existence and his greatest contribution to philosophy. He wrote over 100 treatises. Twenty-one of these were major works, of which sixteen were in medicine.

His most famous work is *The Canon of Medicine* (*Al-Qanun fi' Tibb*), a five-volume medical encyclopedia that collectively contained all the medical knowledge available in the tenth century. It was translated into many languages and was the standard medical textbook in the Islamic world and Europe up to the eighteenth century. The *Canon*, as it is often called, still plays an important role in Unani medicine.

Sir William Osler, the great philosopher of modern medicine, has called the *Canon* "the most famous medical textbook ever written," noting that it remained "a medical bible for a longer time than any other work." Known copies of its translation into Latin, French, Italian, Persian, Turkish, and other languages are preserved in museums around the world.

The Book of Healing (*Kitab al-Shifa*) Ibn Sina's scientific and philosophical encyclopedia was published in 1027 CE. Despite its title, it is not concerned with medicine, but is rather a major work on science and philosophy intended to "cure" or "heal" ignorance of the soul. The book is divided into four parts—logic, natural sciences, mathematics, and metaphysics, and covers a variety of subjects including astronomy, chemistry, earth sciences, psychology, and music.

Another of his treatises, translated into Latin as "Liber Primus Naturalium" played a significant role in the intellectual and philosophical movement that dominated seventeenth- and eighteenth-century Europe. Ibn Sina also wrote Arabic and Persian poems. The last of them is considered a classical beauty. In it he describes the descent of the soul into the body from the higher sphere. He was a unique phenomenon, not only because of his encyclopedic accomplishments in medicine but also due to the versatility of his genius. He is often compared to Aristotle, Leonardo da Vinci, and Goethe.

After a change of rulers, Ibn Sina was imprisoned in the fortress of Fardajan for four months. Subsequent to his release, he moved to Isfahan, where he was received with great respect and esteem. The following years proved the most stable period of his life. He served as the vizier to Ala al-Dawla, the Kakuyid ruler of Isfahan, and accompanied the ruler on many military expeditions. During one of these battles, Ibn Sina experienced a severe case of colic, with which he had suffered throughout his life. He treated himself unsuccessfully and died at the early age of fifty-seven. He was buried in Hamadan.

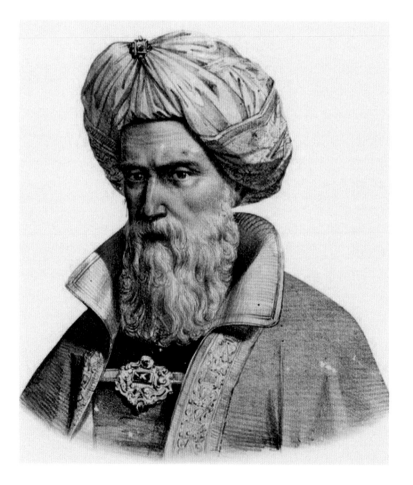

A romanticized engraving of Ibn Sina (Avicenna)

Folios from Ibn Sina's (Avicenna) books

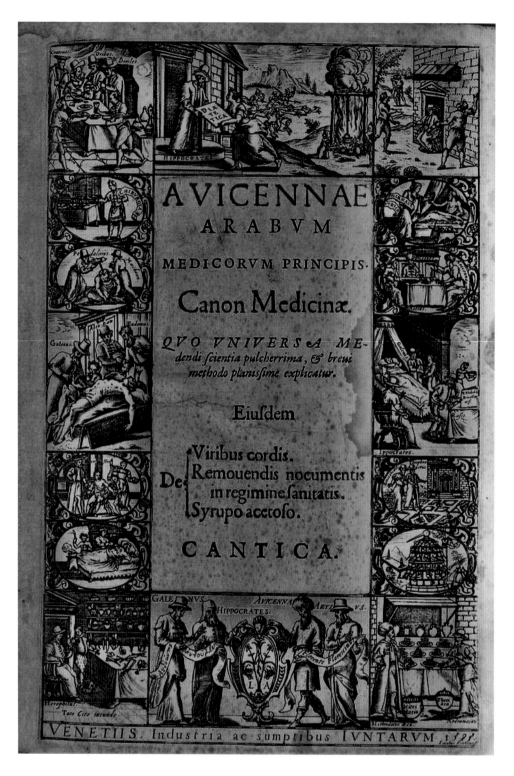

The title page of the original Latin translation of Ibn Sina's

(Avicenna) Qanun fil-tibb(Canon Medicinae)

21. Abul-i-ala Ibn Zuhr (Avenzoar) (1094–1162 CE)

Ibn Zuhr, who was born and died in Seville, Spain, was an Arab physician, surgeon, and poet of medieval Andalusia. One of the most well-respected doctors of his era. He was particularly well-known for his emphasis on a rational and empirical basis for medicine. He belonged to the notable Banu Zuhr family, which had produced six consecutive generations of physicians and many midwives, jurists, poets, and viziers serving the rulers of al-Andalus. Ibn Zuhr started with a religious education, which was customary. At an early age his father, Abul-ala Zuhr tutored him in medicine. His father introduced him to the works of Galen and Hippocrates and had him take the Hippocratic Oath while he was still in his youth.

He started his career as a court physician for the Almoravid empire, a Berber Muslim dynasty centered in Morocco. For an unknown reason he fell out of favor with the ruler and was jailed in Marrakesh in 1140. Seven years later, when Seville was conquered by the Almohad caliphate, he returned to Seville and devoted himself to medical practice.

One of Ibn Zuhr's greatest contributions to medicine was the introduction of animal testing to the experimental method. To confirm that a procedure would work on humans, he first practiced it on animals. The most notable example was his approval and recommendation for tracheostomy, after he performed the procedure on a goat. He was a pioneer in describing many diseases including scabies, otitis media, and pericarditis. Ibn Rushd praised him as the greatest physician since Galen, and the famous Jewish physician-philosopher Maimonides described him as "unique in his age and one of the greatest sages."

One of Ibn Zuhr's major work was *Al-Taysir fil-Mudawat wal-Tadbir* (*Book of Simplification concerning Therapeutics and Diet*). The book was translated into Latin and Hebrew and influenced the development of surgery. He stressed the importance of a practical and sound understanding of anatomy and insisted on a well-supervised and structured surgical training program. He was the first to recognize many diseases and he developed many innovative treatments. He is credited with the first accurate description of esophageal and stomach cancer. He believed in prophylaxis against urinary stone disease and emphasized the importance of dietary management for it. I

His *Kitab al-Iqtisad* (*Book of Moderation*) was a treatise on general therapy with a summary of different diseases, therapeutics, and hygiene. Ibn Zuhr was the first to recommend plastic surgery to alter acquired features such as big noses, thick lips, or crooked teeth.

Kitab al-Aghdiya (*Book of Foods*) is a manual classifying different kinds of foods based on their taste, usefulness, and digestibility as a guideline for healthy living.

Kitab al-Taysir, the last book Ibn Zuhr wrote before his death, was composed as a compendium to Averroes's medical encyclopedia. The two books were later translated into Latin and Hebrew and printed as a single book that remained popular up to the eighteenth century. Ibn Zuhr died in 1162 at the age of sixty-eight in Seville.

22. Muhadhdhab al-Din al-Baghdadi (Ibn Butlan) (1001–1064 CE)

Ibn Butlan was born in Baghdad and died in Antakya, Turkey. An Arab Nestorian Christian physician, he practiced medicine in Baghdad during the Islamic golden age. He traveled to Cairo in 1040 CE to study under Ali Ibn Ridwan, who monopolized the teaching of medicine there. Major differences of opinion led to debates and accusations, and eventually Ibn Ridwan used his influence to drive Ibn Butlan out of Cairo. Ibn Butlan settled in Constantinople but left the city because of a bad plague. Weary of his wanderings and disappointments, he retired to a monastery in Antakya, where he remained as a monk till his death in 1064.

Ibn Butlan is the author of *Taqwim al-Sihhah* (*Maintenance of Health*), best known in the West in its Latin translation, *Tacuinum Sanitatis*. The book dealt with matters of hygiene, dietetics, and exercise. It emphasized the benefits of regular attention to personal physical and mental well-being. The continued popularity and publication of Ibn Butlan's book well into the sixteenth century clearly proves two things: first the importance of preventive medicine, and second the great influence the golden age of Islamic civilization had on early Europe, thereby laying the foundation of modern medicine. He wrote many other books and treatise that did not gain the same popularity.

23. Abdul Walid Ibn Rushd (Averroes) (1126–1198 CE)

Ibn Rushd was born in Cordoba and died in Marrakesh, Morocco. A Muslim Andalusian polymath and jurist, he wrote on many subjects, including philosophy, theology, medicine, astronomy, physics, psychology, mathematics, linguistics, and Islamic jurisprudence and law. He authored more than 100 books and treatises and was known in the Western world as Averroes, the commentator, and the father of rationalism. He argued that scriptural text should be interpreted allegorically if it appears to contradict conclusions reached by reason and philosophy. In the field of medicine, he proposed a new theory on stroke and was the first to identify that the retina is the part of the eye responsible for sensing light. He was also the pioneer in describing the signs and symptoms of Parkinson's disease.

Among his medical books the best-known was *Al-Kulliyat fi al-Tibb* (*The General Principles of Medicine*). Translated into Latin and known as *Colliget*, it was used as a textbook in Europe for centuries. It was a summary of all the medical science available at that time. Another of Ibn Rushd's books, *Al-Taisir*, addressed practical medicine and consisted of excerpts and clinical descriptions of diseases, including serous pericarditis and mediastinal abscess, with which he himself had been afflicted.

In theology, Ibn Rushd upheld the doctrine of divine unity (*tawhid*) and argued that God has seven divine attributes: knowledge, life, power, will, hearing, vision, and speech. He devotes the most attention to the attribute of knowledge and contended that divine knowledge differs from human knowledge because God knows the universe as He created it, while humans know it only through its effects. He further stated that because God created the world, He necessarily knows every part of it in the same way an artist understands his or her work intimately.

Ibn Rushd's philosophical thought created controversies in both the Islamic world and Christendom. The philosophical movement called Averroism was based on the unity of the intellect thesis, which proposed all humans share the same intellect. This belief was declared heretical by Muslims and Christians alike because it contradicts the doctrine of personal immorality. Because of his bold ideas, Ibn Rushd was dismissed from his work and sent to Marrakesh, where he was kept in prison till his death on December 12, 1198.

24. Ali Ibn Ahmad Ibn Hubal (1122–1213 CE)

Ibn Hubal was born in Baghdad and died in Mosul, Iraq. An Arab physician, medical authority, and an accomplished poet. He migrated to Khilat, Turkey, where he became very prosperous in the service of the local ruler, Shah-i-Arman. He later moved to Mardin to serve another lord, Badr al-Din Lu'Lu'. He is best known for his compendium titled *Kitab al-Mukhtarat fi al-Tibb* (*Book of Selections in Medicine*). It was completed in 1165 in Mosul, where Ibn Hubal spent most of his life. This popular medical encyclopedia was largely derived from Ibn Sina's *The Canon* and al-Razi's medical encyclopedia, *Al-Hawi*. Additionally, it drew both on Galen and Ibn Hubal's own personal clinical practice. The work was divided into three main parts, anatomy and general principles, a pharmacopoeia, and a list of maladies arranged according to the affected organs from head to toe. The widely consulted chapter on kidney and bladder stones was translated into multiple languages, including Latin, French, and German. He finally moved to Mosul and unfortunately became blind at the age of seventy-five.

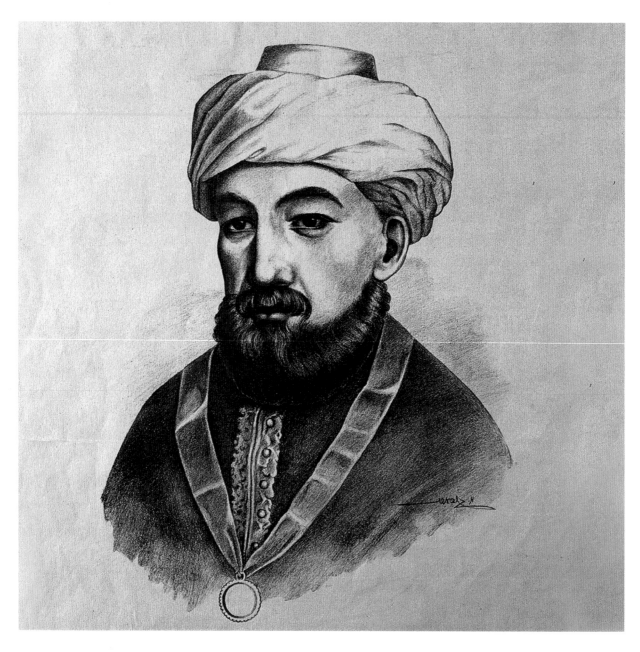

A portrait of Maimonides

THE CONTRIBUTIONS OF ISLAMIC CIVILIZATION TO MEDICINE

25. Moses Ben Maimon (Maimonides) (1135–1204 CE)

Ben Maimon was born in Cordoba and died in Fustat, Egypt. Popularly known as Maimonides, he was a medieval Sephardic Jewish philosopher and one of the most prolific and influential Torah scholars of the Middle Ages. He was also a preeminent astronomer and physician. He was trained in medicine in Cordoba and Fez, Morocco. Gaining widespread recognition, he was appointed court physician to al-Qadi al-Fadil, the chief secretary of the sultan, and later to the sultan Salah ad-Din (Saladin) himself. After the sultan's death, he remained a physician to the Ayyubid dynasty.

In his medical writings, Maimonides described many conditions, including asthma, diabetes hepatitis, and pneumonia. He emphasized moderation in the pursuit of healthy living. Many of his treatises, which became influential for generations of physicians, were based on the makeup and workings of the human body (humorism). He did not blindly accept authority but used his own observation and experience before interpreting works of famous scholars.

Maimonides had an exceptional ability to understand the culture of the patient and respected the patient's autonomy. He devoted most of his time to caring for others. After visiting the sultan's palace he would return home, exhausted and hungry to face a large number of patients waiting at his door. In a letter he wrote, "I would go to heal them and write prescriptions for their illnesses … until the evening … and I would be extremely weak."

Maimonides remains one of the most widely debated Jewish thinkers among modern scholars and is considered an intellectual hero by almost all major movements in modern Judaism. His *Mishneh Torah* is considered by Jews, even today, one of the chief authoritative codifications of Jewish law and ethics.

Of the many medical books and treatise Maimonides authored, the most important, *Regimen Sanitalis* (*Guide to Good Health*), was translated from Arabic to Latin. It was composed by him for Sultan Salah ad-Din's son Sultan al-Afdal. Though many of his prescriptions are obsolete, his advice about public hygiene, preventive medicine. and approach to the patient remain true today.

He wrote ten other medical texts in Arabic, many of which were recently translated into contemporary English, including those addressing asthma, hemorrhoids, poison and their antidotes, and a complete pharmacopeia. The "Oath of Maimonides" is a document about the medical calling and is sometimes recited as a substitute for the Hippocratic Oath.

Maimonides died on December 12, 1204, in Fustat, Egypt and was briefly buried in a synagogue courtyard. Soon afterward, based on his wishes, his remains were exhumed and reburied in Tiberias, on the western shore of the Sea of Galilee.

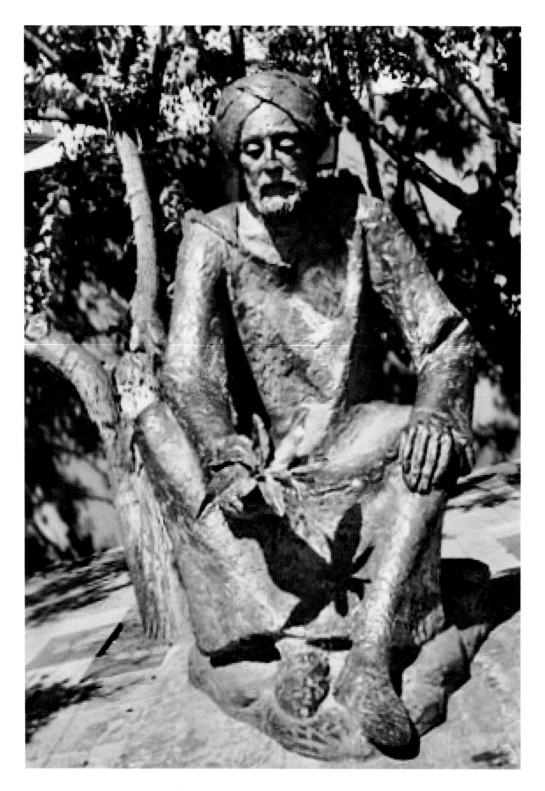

A well-preserved statue of Ibn al-Baitar

THE CONTRIBUTIONS OF ISLAMIC CIVILIZATION TO MEDICINE

26. Abdallah Ibn Ahmad al-Malaqi (Ibn al-Baitar) (1197–1248 CE)

Ibn al-Baitar was born in Malaga, Spain, and died in Damascus, Syria. His name means "son of the veterinarian." An Andalusian Arab physician, botanist, pharmacist, and scientist, he spent his early years in Spain learning botany from a renowned botanist, Abu al-Abbas al-Nabati. Along with his mentor, he was responsible for developing an early scientific method in the testing, description, identification, and therapeutic evaluation of substances used as medicine. He traveled widely as the chief herbalist of the Ayyubid sultan, al-Kamil, through North Africa and then as far as Anatolia, Turkey. In 1227 the Sultan of Damascus appointed him to a similar position. His botanical research extended over a vast area including Arabia and Palestine.

Ibn al-Baitar's largest and most widely read book was *Kitab al-Jami li-Mufradat al-Adwiya wa-l-Aghadhiya* (*Compendium on Simple Medicaments and Foods*). It is a pharmaceutical encyclopedia listing 1,400 plants, foods, and drugs and their uses. Organized alphabetically by the name of the useful plant or plant compound, each entry had a short description, brief remarks by Ibn al-Baitar and reports of previous authors. In the modern printed Arabic version, the book is more than 900 pages long. It was published in full in translation into German and French.

Ibn al-Baitar's second book, *Kitab al-Mughnifi al-Adwiya al-Mufrada*, is an encyclopedia of Islamic medicine that incorporates his knowledge of plants used for the treatment of various ailments, including diseases involving the head, eye, ear, etc. His works were widely translated and remained a key resource for scientists and physicians over the next several centuries, falling into disuse only in the late eighteenth and early nineteenth centuries. Ibn al-Baitar died in 1248 at the early age of fifty-one.

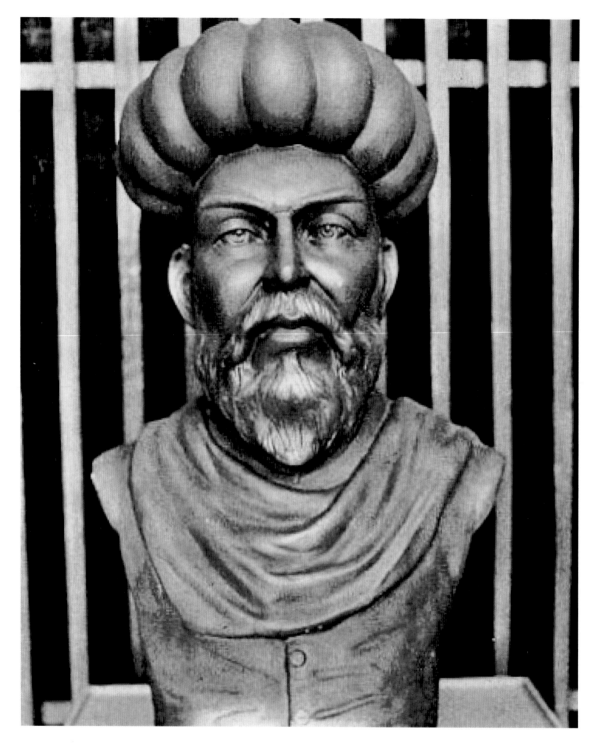

A statue of Ibn al-Nafis

THE CONTRIBUTIONS OF ISLAMIC CIVILIZATION TO MEDICINE

27. Ala-al-Din Abu al-Hassan Ali Ibn al-Nafis (1213–1288 CE)

Ibn al-Nafis was born in Damascus and died in Cairo, Egypt. An Arab polymath, whose areas of interest included medicine, surgery, physiology, anatomy, biology, Islamic studies, jurisprudence, and philosophy.

He was known for describing the pulmonary circulation of blood and has been called the father of circulatory physiology. As an early anatomist, Ibn al-Nafis performed human dissections, leading to several important discoveries in the fields of anatomy and physiology. Apart from medicine, Ibn al-Nafis was also a philosopher, linguist, and historian and was considered an expert on the Shafai' school of jurisprudence.

Starting at the age of sixteen, Ibn al-Nafis studied medicine for ten years at Nuri Hospital in Damascus. In 1236 CE, along with some of his colleagues, he moved to Egypt under the Ayyubid sultan, al-Kamil. There he was appointed chief physician at al-Naseri Hospital, originally established by Salah ad-Din, the founder of the Ayyubid dynasty.

One of Ibn al-Nafis's most notable students was the famous Christian physician Ibn al-Quff. During this era, the medical profession was severely affected by the Mongol Tartar invasion and destruction of Baghdad. Islamic culture was also declining in Spain, making Cairo and Damascus the centers of medical education and prestige. With the rise of the Mamluk dynasty, Ibn al-Nafis was appointed the personal physician of Sultan Abu al-Futuh and other prominent political leaders. He continued his career in Cairo for the rest of his life. At the age of seventy-four Ibn al-Nafis was appointed the first chief physician of al-Mansuri Hospital, and in 1284 he became the dean of the school of medicine. He died in Cairo on December 17, 1288.

Ibn al-Nafis wrote several books and commentaries on different topics, including medicine, law, philosophy, theology, grammar, and the environment. The most voluminous of his books on medicine is *Al-Shamil fi al-Tibb* (*The Comprehensive Book of Medicine*). Even though Ibn al-Nafis completed only 80 volumes of the planned 300-volume encyclopedia, the work is considered one of the largest medical encyclopedias ever written by one person. It gave a complete summary of all the medical knowledge the Islamic world possessed at that time. Extant manuscripts of this work are cataloged in many libraries around the world, including Cambridge University Library and Lane Medical Library at Stanford University in California.

Another of Ibn al-Nafis's famous works was *Sharha Tashrih al-Qanun* (*Commentary on Anatomy in Book I and II of Ibn Sina's Kitab al-Qanun*). Ibn al-Nafis published it when he was twenty-nine years old. The book remains of great interest today, because it contains several ground-breaking contributions to our understanding of the pulmonary circulation, including his prediction of the pulmonary capillaries four centuries before their discovery by the Italian Marcello Malpighi. Besides the discussion of anatomy and physiology, what distinguishes the book most is the confident language Ibn al-Nafis used throughout the text and his boldness in challenging the most established medical authorities of the time including Galen and Ibn Sina.

In describing pulmonary, coronary, and capillary circulation, Ibn al-Nafis postulated that nutrients for the heart are extracted from the coronary arteries. He also clarified the concept of the pulse. "The pulse" he wrote, "is a direct result of the heartbeat; the arteries contract when the heart expands and expand when the heart contracts." He authored several books on surgery, urology, and metabolism.

A manuscript of Ibn al-Nafis's concerning Hippocrates's *On the Nature of Man* is preserved by the US National Library of Medicine, the world's largest medical library. Ibn al-Nafis also composed the first Arabic commentary on Hippocrates's *Epidemics*. In it Ibn al-Nafis described the method of locating the origin of an outbreak, which Dr. John Snow used in 1854 to trace the source of a cholera outbreak in Soho, London.

Ibn al-Nafis's mastery of the medical sciences, his prolific writings, and his image as a devout religious scholar left a positive impression on later Muslim biographers and historians, who described him as the greatest physician of his time, a second Ibn Sina.

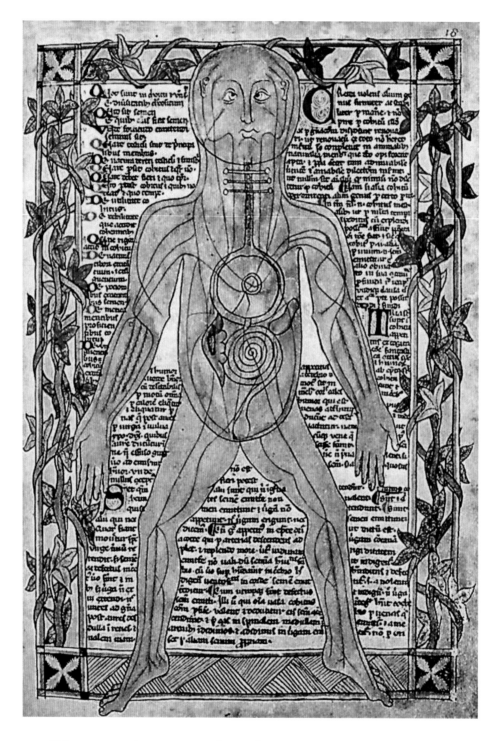

Diagrammatic anatomy of circulation as perceived by al-Nafis

28. Amin ud-Daula Farj Ibn al-Quff (1233–1286 CE)

Ibn al-Quff was born in Kerak, Jordan, and died in Damascus. A Melkite Christian Arab physician and surgeon, he was the author of the earliest and largest medieval Arabic treatise intended solely for surgeons. When he was young, his family moved to Syria, where he was introduced to medical studies.

He acquired considerable medical knowledge by reading and spent large amounts of time meditating on the material. As he began to practice, his reputation began to spread across the empire as a physician sincerely caring for his patients and conducting his work with great honesty. In Damascus, he extended his knowledge with the study of metaphysics, philosophy, the natural sciences, and mathematics. Having established himself as a well-educated physician and surgeon, he was appointed to a high position in the army and stationed in Jordan, where he was born.

During this time, because he wrote many books and taught medicine, Ibn al-Quff became better known as a writer and educator than as a doctor. He completed ten books, of which seven are known to exist today, either in complete form or in fragments.

Ibn al-Quff's most famous work, *Kitab al-Umda fi 'l-giraha* (*Basics in the Art of Surgery*), was by far the largest Arabic text on surgery published during the entire medieval period. It was a general medical manual covering anatomy, medical care with drugs, and surgical care, with a special emphasis on wounds and tumors. He explained the connections between arteries, veins, capillaries, and valves more than three centuries before the invention of the microscope. His first medical encyclopedia, *Al-Shafi al-Tibb* (*The Comprehensive Book of the Healing Arts*) was completed before he turned forty years old. His sixty-volume book on preventive medicine and advice for preserving health was published a few years later in 1272 CE.

Several of his books were commentaries on the works of Hippocrates and Ibn Sina. His book, *Zubad al-Tabib*, was wholly devoted to advice for practicing physicians. Ibn al-Quff was the first to mention the word *anesthetic* in Arabic. He carefully explained the involvement of the physician in providing mixtures of drugs to prevent pain during surgical procedures. The recommended methods of administering these drugs were inhalation, ingestion, and rectal suppositories. The drugs used included opium, mandrake, cannabis, and belladonna. Ibn al-Quff died in 1286 in Damascus at the early age of fifty-three.

29. Mansur Ibn Yusuf Ibn Ilyas (1380–1422 CE)

Ibn Ilyas was born and died in Shiraz, Persia. A late fourteenth-century anatomist and physician, he came from a wealthy, educated, and respected family. After studying in a traditional Persian school, he left Shiraz and traveled to many other cities, including Tabriz, which was known for its rich scientific background.

Ibn Iyas's most famous work was *Tashrih-i Mansuri* (*The Anatomy of the Human Body*), believed to be the first illustrated anatomical manuscript containing two-dimensional pictures of the human body in full-color. Composed in Persian, this fourteenth-century treatise is organized into five sections on the skeleton, nerves, muscles, veins, and arteries. Each illustration is a full-page diagram, and the final chapter includes an image of a pregnant woman delivering a breech baby. As Professor Eamonn Gearon of Johns Hopkins University remarked "Although he is virtually unknown in the west today, his most famous work is housed in the world's largest medical library: the U.S. National Library of Medicine in Bethesda, Maryland." Ibn Ilyas's illustrations were copied and notated in many other languages and were often used in other manuscripts for at least two centuries.

His other famous book was *Kifaya-yi Mansuri* (*A Synopsis of General Medicine*). Both of these major medical works as well as a medical encyclopedia are dedicated to the ruler of the Persian province of Fars, Prince Pir Mohammad Bahador Khan, the grandson of Tamerlane. In most of his writing, Ibn Ilyas engaged in controversial topics, making references to the works of Aristotle, Hippocrates, al-Razi, and Ibn Sina. Since a considerable portion of his work was dedicated to the central and peripheral nervous systems, Ibn Ilyas is considered the father of neuroanatomy.

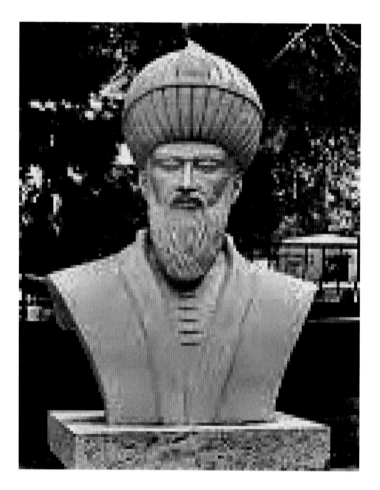

A statue of Sabuncuoglu Serafeddin

30. Sabuncuoglu Serafeddin (CE 1385–1468)

Serafeddin was born and died in Amasya, Turkey. A fifteenth-century Ottoman Turkish physician and surgeon, he started his medical studies at the age of seventeen. His grandfather Mevlana el-Kac Ilyas Celebi was the chief physician of Ottoman Sultan Mehmed I. He learned medicine at Amasya Hospital, where he worked and practiced for fourteen years. The Hospital was built in the early period of the Ottoman Empire, in 1308, and served the district of Amasya, a center for commerce, culture, and the arts. After this Serafeddin moved to Istanbul, where he authored most of his writings, finally returning to Amasya, where he died in 1468.

Serafeddin's first major work was the translation and addition to a medical encyclopedia written by Zayn al-Din Gorgani, *Akrabazin* (*Pharmacology*). He then authored *Cerrhiyyetu'l-Haniyye* (*Imperial Surgery*), the first illustrated surgical atlas to be published and the last major medical encyclopedia from the Islamic golden age. This work, mainly based on al-Zahrawi's *Al-Tasrif*, introduced many innovations. He presented the book to Sultan Mehmed II, better known as Mehmed the Conqueror. The book was written in Turkish, primarily for medical students, and had miniatures depicting surgical operations. Three copies of the book exist in their original form—two at the Millet Library in Istanbul and one at the Bibliothèque Nationale in Paris.

Serafeddin's third work to survive the ages was *Mucerrebname* (*On Attempt*), a pharmacological guide that offers special recipes for specific diseases. One interesting part of this book treats his own experiences with drugs applied to himself, other human beings, and sometimes animals. Ottoman physicians used his books as a guide for centuries and Sabuncuoglu Serafeddin became a prominent name in the history of Turkish medicine. The university hospital in Amasya and the neighborhood where he was born have been named after him.

Serafeddin was the first to describe a technique for the drainage of hydrocephalus. He also introduced axial traction for spinal surgery. He pioneered the usage of wooden splints after hand surgery. In the field of obstetrics, he recommended the use of herbals to promote faster delivery of the fetus. He recommended certain herbs and cauterization of the forehead for treatment of epilepsy. Having an awareness of pathogens causing sepsis, he wore surgical attire and used wine and olive oil as antiseptics.

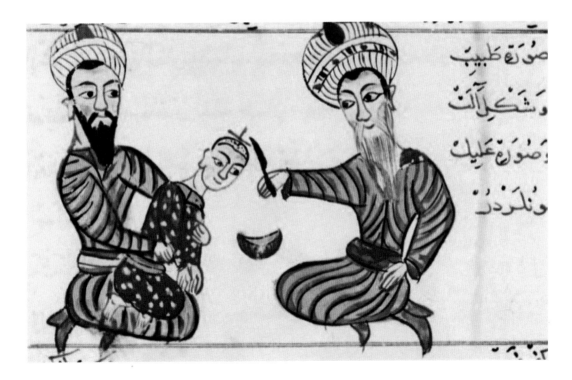

Draining fluid from a child with hydrocephalus

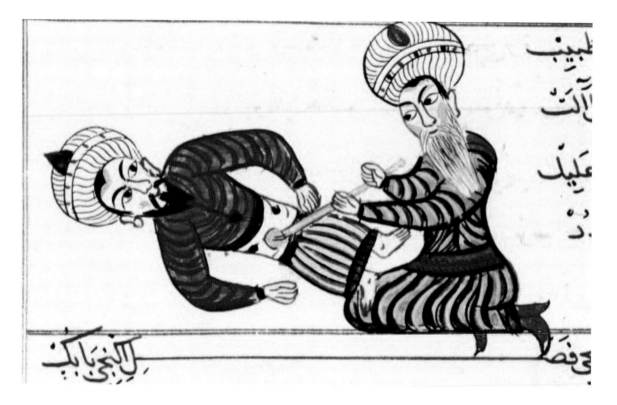

Draining fluid from the abdominal cavity in a patient suffering from dropsy

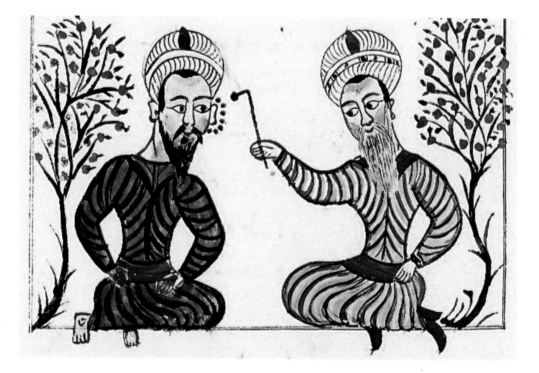

Treating earache

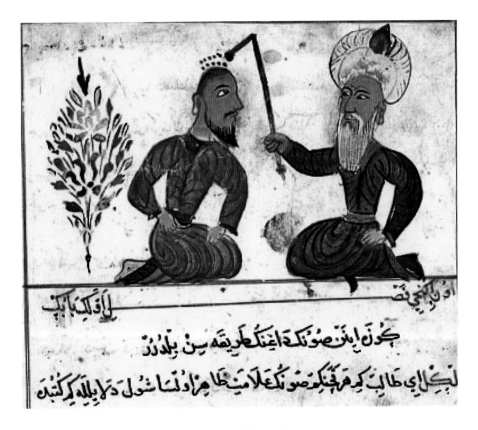

Treating Migraine

Miniatures depicting common procedures from the Medical Atlas of Imperial Surgery
by Subuncuoglu Serefeddin 1466 CE

31. Dawud Ibn Umar al-Antaki (1543–1599 CE)

Al-Antaki was born to a Christian family in Antioch, Turkey, and died in Makkah, Saudi Arabia. A blind Syrian Muslim physician and pharmacist, he spent most of his active years in Cairo, Egypt. Seminal Western historian of Arabic medicine Lucien Leclerc (1876) called al-Antaki "dernier représentant de la médecine arabe" (the last great representative of Arabian medicine). Despite having been born blind, al-Antaki traveled extensively in the Islamic empire. He lived in Damascus and Cairo and died while living in Makkah in 1599.

Among al-Antaki's writings, the most famous is *Tadhkira uli al-albab wa'l-Jami' li al-ajab al-ujab (A Reminder to Intellectuals and a Collection of the Wonder of Wonders)*. The book is as a medical compendium covering both illness and remedies. Chapter I concerns general medical principles, Chapter II deals with the basic rules of preparing drugs, and Chapters III and IV list diseases in alphabetical order with their symptoms, therapies, and simple and compound remedies and cures. A whole section of *Tadhkira* deals with coffee and was translated by Edward Pococke in 1659 with the title "The nature of the drink Kauhi, of Coffee, and the berry of which it is made described by an Arabian physician." An original copy is now in the Bodleian Library while a copy dated 1838 is in the Museum of Islamic Art in Doha, Qatar.

Other works by al-Antaki are also well known, including *Tadhkir al-Qabb (A Reminder of All Things)*, a three-part book dealing with herbal medicines that includes descriptions of over 3,000 medicinal and aromatic plants. His *Book of Precious Kohl for the Evacuation of the President's Eyes* is an explanation of Ibn Sina's poem. Al-Antaki also wrote three books on astronomy, some works on logic, and a book on psychiatry that contains hadiths offering medical advice. In 1598 CE al-Antaki made a pilgrimage to Makkah. He decided to stay on and passed away a year later.

CHAPTER 4:

The Islamic Principles of Hygiene as Practiced by Muhammad Bin Abdullah (PBUH)

Ramzi Mohammad, MSc, PhD

Introduction

Islam places immense emphasis on cleanliness. The Prophet Muhammad's (PBUH) hygiene practices were far ahead of his time. The guidelines he laid out over 1,440 years ago taught people how to purify themselves, preserve their health, implement self-care, prevent illness, and maintain freshness and beauty in both the personal and public spheres. This knowledge was not only adopted globally but it raised the standards of civilization and are completely in line with the highest qualities of cleanliness today.

Cleanliness Is Half of Faith

Cleanliness is required in Islam. So much so, that the Prophet Muhammad (PBUH) declared that "cleanliness is half of faith." While humankind generally considers cleanliness a revered trait, Islam insists on it. Muslims throughout the world have incredibly high standards of personal hygiene. Prayers cannot even be performed unless the body is in a state of purity. Islam teaches the importance of both physical and spiritual cleanliness. The Holy Quran, the book of Islam, instructs the faithful to keep clean. God states that He "loves those who turn to Him in repentance, and He loves those who keep themselves pure and clean" (Quran 2:222).

Not only is personal hygiene always emphasized, but certain aspects are compulsory. Ritual washing is a prerequisite to prayer. This is a regular form of cleanliness that Muslims incorporate into their lives multiple times every day. Ritual bathing is also required. Keeping one's body, clothes, home, and space clean is the responsibility of every capable person. Removing dirt or impurities that may exist in various parts of the body such as teeth, nails, nose, armpits, and the pubic area is also prescribed to maintain basic conditions of cleanliness. Muslims are required to take care of their personal hygiene, ensuring they are well groomed, smell nice, and look refined. This not only applies to their bodies but to their environments, such as their homes, schools, workplaces, healthcare centers, mosques, and all other surroundings.

Ritual Wash

Purity is vital to prayer. The Arabic word for purity is *tahara*, which means to be free from filth—both physical and spiritual. Spiritual purity means being free from sin and idolatry and requires sincere belief in the Oneness of God. Before a person stands before God in the special connection that is prayer, he must ensure his heart is free from sin, arrogance, and hypocrisy. He must also make sure he is clean from physical impurities. Water can be used to achieve this. "O you who believe! When you intend to offer the prayer, wash your faces and your hands up to the elbows, wipe your heads, and wash your feet up to the ankles. If you are in a state of Janaba (e.g., had sexual discharge) purify yourself" (Quran 5:6).

Prior to prayer, a person must make sure he is in a state of cleanliness. He does this by performing a ritual wash called *wudu* or a full bath called *ghusl*. *Wudu* rids the body of minor impurities while *ghusl* cleanses the body of major ones. *Ghusl* must be performed after sexual intercourse or any sexual activity that releases bodily fluids. *Ghusl* is also performed at the completion of a woman's menstrual period or postpartum bleeding. The cleansing ritual of *wudu* includes washing the hands, rinsing both mouth and nose, washing the face, washing the arms up to the elbows, wiping the head, washing the ears, including behind them, and washing the feet, including the ankle. Prophet Muhammad (PBUH) taught people to do this in an environmentally friendly manner. He recommended using as little water as necessary to complete the *wudu* correctly. He forbade wastefulness or harm of any kind. His traditions improve overall health and well-being. Islam is a holistic religion tailored to the natural needs of humankind.

Circumcision

Circumcision is obligatory for males providing there is no harm to them. This makes it easier to keep the genitals clean from traces of urine, dirt, or other impurities.

Cutting Nails

The reason for keeping the nails short is hygiene. Dirt and bacteria can easily be trapped under the nails and passed on to others, especially when preparing food or in a medical environment. Having unkempt fingernails or toenails is unhealthy and unhygienic.

Hair Care

Prophet Muhammad (PBUH) made clear to his followers that they should take care of their hair, keeping it clean, washed, well groomed, and smelling nice. He would apply nourishing oil in his hair to keep it healthy, fresh, shiny, and smelling good. He advised men to trim their mustaches and tend to their beards.

Armpit and Pubic Hair

Removing the hair from the armpits makes it easier to clean this area of the body where sweat and dirt may collect. This prevents growth of bacteria or a bad smell. Removing pubic hair is obligatory to keep clean; therefore, the removal of pubic hair is instructed. Muslims are encouraged to keep their genital area and underwear as clean as possible. Moreover, if this area is not cleaned properly, it can lead to health issues. Muslim homes often have water hoses installed next to the toilet or water jugs available to ease cleanliness.

Oral Care

Islam emphasizes oral hygiene. Prophet Muhammad [PBUH] revolutionized dental care. He taught his followers the significance of cleaning their teeth. He used a toothbrush called a *miswak*, a natural twig fortified with minerals that cleans the teeth, prevents the gums from bleeding, kills bacteria, and freshens breath. Prophet Muhammad said, "Use *miswak*, for it purifies the mouth and pleases the Lord," and "Had it not been for fear of making things too difficult for my nation, I would have instructed them to clean their teeth with *miswak* before every prayer."

Islamic Hygiene to Prevent Disease

Many recommendations concerning personal hygiene and overall cleanliness of the environment were followed during Islamic civilization: keeping clothes clean, washing one's mouth and hands before and after a meal, keeping food and water covered, using fragrance or perfume, combing, and using oil on the hair, keeping homes and roads clean, covering the face when coughing or sneezing, maintaining social distance, and making loud noises or raising voices.

As the coronavirus has clearly portrayed, the importance of handwashing, social distancing, covering the mouth and nose, and cleanliness cannot be underestimated. Implementing these Islamic guidelines keeps diseases and viruses at bay. Regular and thorough handwashing has proven effective in preventing infection. Before every prayer, at least five times a day, Muslims perform the mandatory *wudu*, which includes washing the hands three times each. Islam's emphasis on cleanliness aligns with anti-pandemic rules and strongly supports individuals' ability to protect themselves from fatal viruses. It is documented that when Prophet Muhammad (PBUH) sneezed, he would cover his face with his hand or with his garment and muffle the sound with it. Most of his teachings came after he had been ordained to be a prophet. God, the creator of the heavens and earth, knows what is best for mankind. God states in the Quran, "We have not sent you except that you are a mercy to the worlds."

Islamic Hygienic Practices in History

Societies quickly learned Islamic teachings and implemented them into their own social norms, adopting everything from implementing daily habits to creating new infrastructure and facilities to support them. The

Muslims created public baths while these facilities were often neglected in the rest of the world. To supply its half a million inhabitants with running water, Cordoba in Muslim Spain had 300 public baths known as *hammams*. Turkish baths, which were not popular across Europe, followed this tradition. Islamic Cordoba also showcased operative streetlights and running water, while people around the globe were ignorant of such advancements.

Since beauty salons were common in Muslim Spain (Andalusia), famous Muslim physician al-Zahrawi devoted a complete chapter to cosmetics in his medical encyclopedia, *al-Tasrif*. This included underarm deodorants, hair-removing sticks, hand lotions, hair dyes, and hair relaxers. He even mentioned the benefits of sunscreen and described it beneficial ingredients. Al-Kindi, a Muslim Iraqi scholar and scientist, wrote a book on perfumes, recipes for fragrant oils, creams, and scented waters, making an immense contribution to the world of fragrance. More than 1,000 years ago the Muslim musician Ziryab introduced toothpaste in Spain.

Conclusion

The principles of hygiene developed and practiced during the era of Islamic civilization was based on divine wisdom and the life and practices of Prophet Mohammad (PBUH).

CHAPTER 5:

Principles and Development of Islamic Medical Ethics: A Historical Account

Hossam Fadel, MD, PhD, FACOG

Editorial Note: Throughout this article although the male pronouns "he/his" are used it refers to both male and female genders.

Introduction

Ethics, which represents manners and morals, initially was limited to individuals' personal characters. As societies developed and individuals were grouped into professions, the concept of ethics expanded to include certain codes of behavior for the different professions, most notably the medical profession. Healthcare essentially entails direct and personal interaction with other individuals when they need help and are in emotional as well as physical distress.

The Quran is replete with verses describing the characters and morals that are pleasing to God. Many of the Prophet Muhammad's (PBUH) sayings guide Muslims to live a virtuous life. Muslims are required to abide by certain behavior, outlined in Shariah that allows for a peaceful and just society. In addition, many of the Prophet's traditions (*ahadith*) discuss health and disease and encourage pursuing a cure through available spiritual and natural medications, as well as by seeking the help of a qualified physician (*hakim*). Ethics is mainly guided by these divine rules and prophetic guidance.

With significant advances in medicine have come many unprecedented modes of treatment and hitherto unknown techniques and procedures. These require new opinions on how to tackle these and on which ones are acceptable from the Islamic point of view. Ethics has evolved. In addition to the general moral principles applicable to all Muslims, the medical discipline requires studying all new issues and deciding on their juristic implications. This is the scope of Islamic medical ethics. Further, medical progress depends on research—both scientific and clinical. The latter often involves experimentation on humans, which raises another subset of ethics.

In this chapter I will discuss the concept of disease and cure in Islam. Then I will explore the development of ethics from the past to the current times specifically in relation to Islamic guidelines. I will discuss its principles and how new rulings are or can be made. I will also address the importance of clinical research and the special ethical issues it raises, and the importance of oaths for physicians and their development from antiquity till the present.

Concept of Disease and Cure

Muslims believe God controls all events. All difficulties, including disease, are ordained by God. We also believe cure is from God. "When I get sick, He is the One that cures me"[1] Doctors and medications are but tools in God's hand. The doctor, despite being outstanding and expert in his field, can do nothing without God's will and consent.

Muslims also believe we need to actively seek cures. The Prophet Muhammad (PBUH) said, "There is a remedy for every malady except death from old age and when the remedy is applied to the disease it is cured with the permission of God, the exalted and Glorious."[2] He commanded us to look for the cure: "God has sent down both the disease and the cure. He has appointed a cure for every disease, except old age, so treat yourselves but do not use anything unlawful."[3] "God did not make your recovery from illnesses with what He otherwise made forbidden."[4]

The Prophet (PBUH) told us to seek the most experienced and qualified healer. He cautioned us about those who proclaim they are healers but have no experience. "Whoever claims to be a physician though unknown to such a profession is subject to personal liability. He must pay compensation for whatever damage he may cause."[5]

He also encouraged us to visit the sick and stressed the spiritual merits of such a visit, explaining that it contributes to the well-being of the patient. He recommended that the visit be after the third day, when it appears to be a serious illness (not a simple flu). The visit needs to be short and should include words of encouragement and supplication. "Feed the hungry, visit the sick and set free the captives."[6]

Medical liability is enshrined in Islamic law and divided according to different situations.[7] A physician may be highly trained, adhering to the ethics of the profession and performing his services according to the rules, and, despite that, according to divine will, the patient may suffer from complications. In such cases, all Muslim jurists agree the physician will not be liable. The loss will be attributed to an act of God. In the case of an impostor or an ignorant person, if the patient knew his attendant was not a physician and yet consented

---

1. Glorious Quran: Chapter 26, verse 80.

2. Sahih Muslim, Hadith 5466.

3. Sunan Abī Dāwūd. Kitāb al-ṭibb. Bāb fī al-adwiya al-makrūha. Hadith no. 3874. muhaddith.org.

4. Sahih Bukhari (in Medicine of the Prophet, p. 113.

5. Abu dawud, Ibn Maja Medicine of the Prophet, p. 113.

6. Natural healing with the Medicine of the Prophet Ibn Qayyim al-Jawziyya Translation and emendation by Muhammad al-Akili Pearl Publishing House Philadelphia, USA 1993, p. 98.

7. Arawi. T J.Islam.Med.Assn 2010;42:111.

to his treatment, then, again, the physician will not be liable for injury or loss. However, if the patient unsuspectingly thinks the person offering his services is a physician or if the latter convinces the patient by implied presentation or coercion, then the physician will be liable.

If the physician is experienced and performs the services according to the rules but by an unintentional accident causes an injury, then he is not liable. A well-trained physician who attempts his best but still reached a wrong diagnosis or gave the wrong medication will be liable. In this case, the compensation may be given by the physician but could also be paid by the Muslim treasury (*bait-ul-mal*). A well-trained physician who performs a procedure on a minor or a mentally incompetent individual without proper consent from the family will be liable for any loss. However, some scholars would withhold compensation from the physician if he performed the procedure with the consent of the minor or the mentally incompetent patient or as a charitable act (no compensation).

The Ethics (*Akhlaq*) of the Muslim Physician

Ethics is derived from the Greek word *ethikos*, which in turn is derived from the root word *ethos*, meaning customs, norms, or manners. The Arabic word for it is *akhlaqiyyat* (morals or manners). The importance of a physician's good character has been expressed from antiquity. Aristotle believed a virtuous life is at the same time the best, the most noble, and the most pleasant. According to the Qur'an, virtue is not innate at birth but comes about because of habituation. It is a voluntary and purposeful habit that eventually becomes second nature.[8]

In the West ethics evolved in the recent past as a distinct discipline to deal with issues of moral character. In Islam this was not dealt with as separate because it is part and parcel of Islamic teachings. Islam emphasizes virtue (good character/manners/morals). It offers a moral order in which good and evil can be distinguished as these are identified clearly in the Quran and Sunnah. Ethical and moral behavior is described as piety (*taqwa*) and good deeds (*'amal salih*). Observing what is essentially good (*ma'ruf*) and virtuous (*birr*) is an obligation on all Muslims. However, special attention has been paid to those who practice the healing art. Physicians, as they deal with the most honored of God's creation (human beings), especially when they are most vulnerable, should have higher moral standards than the average person. The following is a sample of moral values mentioned in the Quran and Sunnah.

The first verse of the Quran truly encompasses these teachings. "Surely Allah enjoins justice, kindness and doing of good, to kith and kin, and forbids all that is shameful, evil and oppressive. He exhorts you so that you may be mindful."[9]

---

8. The Glorious Quran Chapter 16, verse 90.
9. The Glorious Quran 68, verse 4.

The Quran describes the Prophet Muhammad (PBUH): "And surely you have sublime morals."[10] The Prophet said, "I was sent to complete the best of *akhlaq* (good or moral manners, morality)."[11] "The best among you are those who have the best manners and character."[12]

Muslims are ordered to emulate the Prophet in his behavior and character. The Quran says, "You have indeed in the Messenger of Allah a beautiful pattern (of conduct) for any one whose hope is in Allah and the Final Day."[13] "And for such as had entertained the fear of standing before their Lord's (tribunal) and had restrained (their) soul from lower desires, their abode will be the Garden (Heaven, Paradise)."[14]

Other verses read as follows: "And cover not Truth with falsehood, nor conceal the Truth when you know (what it is)."[15] "Swell not your cheek (for pride) at men. Nor walk in insolence through the earth: For God loves not any arrogant boaster."[16] The Prophet (PBUH) said, "And he who brings the truth and he who confirms (and supports) it—such are the men who are the righteous."[17] "The signs of a hypocrite are three: Whenever he speaks, he tells a lie; and whenever he promises, he breaks his promise; and whenever he is entrusted, he betrays (proves to be dishonest)."[18] "God will not look, on the Day of Resurrection, at a person who drags his *izār* (garment) [behind him] out of pride and arrogance."[19] "The strong is not the one who overcomes the people by his strength, but the strong is the one who controls himself while in anger."[20] "Whoever is not merciful to others will not be treated mercifully."[21]

The physician should not abuse his status for monetary gain. He should avoid all wrongdoing and should not mislead his patients. He must control his desire and should be humble, curtail arrogance, and not lie or waste resources. He should keep patient information confidential and should not make fun of the patient. He must show tolerance, patience, honesty, kindness, and mercy while avoiding pride and anger. Physicians should treat all patients kindly whether they are rich or poor. The Prophet said, "The worst people in the sight

10. Hadith I came to complete best morals.

11. Sahīh Al-Bukhārī. Kitāb al-adab. Bāb husn al-khuluq wal-sakhā' wa mā yukrahu min al-bukhl. Hadith no. 5688. Available from muhaddith.org.

12. The Glorious Quran Chapter 26, Verse 80.

13. The Glorious Quran Chapter 79, verse 40.

14. The Glorious Quran Chapter 2, verse 42.

15. The Glorious Quran Chapter 31, verse 18.

16. The Glorious Quran Chapter 39, verse 33.

17. Sahīh Al-Bukhārī. Kitāb al-libās. Bāb man jarra thawbahu min al-khayulā'. Hadith no. 5451. Available from muhaddith.org.

18. Sahīh al-Bukhārī. Kitāb al-adab. Bāb al-hadhar min al-ghadab. Hadith no. 5763. Available from muhaddith.org.

19. Sahīh al-Bukhārī. Kitāb al-adab. Bāb al-rahmah al-walad wa taqbīlihi wa mu'ānaqatihi. Hadith no.5651.available from muhaddith.org.

20. Sahīh al-Bukhārī. Kitāb al-adab. Bāb mā qīl fi thī al-wajhayn. Hadith no. 5711. Available from muhaddith.org.

21. Adab al-Tabib by Ishaq Ibn Aly al-Ruhawi.???? Marizy Sa'aid Marizy A'ssiry, First ed., Published by King Faisal Center for Islamic Research and Studies, Riyad, Kingdom of Saudi Arabia, 1992, p. 24.(Arabic) إسحاق بن علي الرهاوي مرزين سعيد مرزين عسيري

of God on the Day of Resurrection will be the double-faced people who appear to some people with one face and to other people with another face."[22]

Historical Background

Hippocrates wrote about the moral character of physicians, but early Muslim scholars were the first to dedicate complete books to the subject. Al-Razi wrote a companion book to *Kitab al-Mansuri* dedicated to the reformation of the character of the physician, entitled *al-Tibb al-Ruhani* (*Spiritual Medicine*). In this work he details how a physician can elevate his character by controlling his passions and casting away vices. Yuhanna Ibn Masaweh wrote a book on the same subject, but both these books were lost. The first book that survived is that of Ishaq Ibn Ali al-Ruhawi, *Adab al-Tabib* (*The Ethics of the Physician*). Al-Ruhawi lived around 854–893 CE. An English translation of a manuscript found in Istanbul by Martin Levey has been published. The book is divided into twenty chapters. The following is a synopsis of the Arabic version of the book.[23]

The medical profession is the most noble of professions. The physician who seeks the profession should do that for its sake—that is, to benefit people—not just for earning a living. This will provide permanent satisfaction and joy in addition to a good living. He will have a nice reputation and great remembrance from the people and will be close to God and His pleasure. Not everyone can learn to be a physician. Only those who are of good character and can endure extensve studies and continue the process of learning should enter this profession. In other professions mistakes can be corrected without loss of health or life.

Physicians must be tested before they are allowed to practice, with emphasis on both the theoretical (basic sciences) and practical aspects (technical skills). The physician should be skilled in eliciting symptoms and in looking for signs of disease. He should use a pharmacist he trusts. He should be familiar with the preparation of medications, whether simple or complex, and whether they deteriorate in efficacy or become harmful over time.

The physician should encourage patients or his helpers to be frank with him when mishaps happen such as errors in the use of medications or the preparation of food, or not following his instructions, so the physician can try to fix what went wrong in time to avoid complications. Physicians should consult with each other if needed.

Al-Ruhawi stressed the good moral character of the physician. "He should not be envious, hateful, greedy, nor arrogant. He should be forgiving, kind, humble, thankful, and delighted to be complimented." He cautions physicians against praising of evil ones, or disdain of others, as long as he is doing the right thing.

The physician should take care of his own hygiene and physical appearance. He should always be clean, be sure he has no mouth or body odor, while also observing his dietary habits. He should cut his nails and extra hair on his head and face. It is not polite of him to expectorate, yawn, or stretch himself in public. The physician must guard his five senses. No foul word should be heard from him. He must protect his sight, not

---

22. Adab al-Tabib Transactions of the Amer Philosophical Society Vol 57, part 3,1967 Medical Ethics of Medieval Islam with special Reference to Al-Ruhawi's Practical Ethics of the Physician Translated by Martin Levey Zikria, B A . J Islam Med Assn, 1981;13:79–81.

23. Tahthib al-al-Akhlaq and Tathir al-A'araq by Aby Ahmad Ibn Mohammad Ibn Miskaweyh. Published by the Egyptian Hussainiyyah Printing company, Cairo, Egypt, 1329 H 1911 AC. Available at the American University, Cairo, Egypt (Arabic).

beholding anything vile unless it is necessary. He should not listen to illiterate people or to the statements of the wicked. He should instead frequent assemblies of the virtuous, lettered and learned.

The physician must take care of their outfit. They must be clean and be garments of beauty, especially when he is near people of status. The physician should follow a strict schedule in his daily activities, including a limited time of sleep. He should divide his day between prayer, remembrance, thanking God, studying, and visiting patients both at their homes and in his office. The physician must be just and merciful to the weak and the poor. It is not correct for the physician to earn property by trade since that holds him back from science. It is in the best interest of the physician to avoid play and playthings so he may not become weak-minded and silly. Flattery is not fitting for the physician since it is of the morals of the crowd. Envy is not good for the physician since it causes him to fall from his position.

The physician must be thankful to God for His bounty and sincere in worship. Similarly, nice people should honor and give due respect to physicians. It is bad that when a person is sick, he asks for help from God and from a physician, but once he is cured he does not thank God appropriately and is unkind to the physician. Some patients hate physicians because they tend to advise them against indulgence in vices and other pleasures.

Physicians must prepare themselves for getting old, weak, or incapacitated by paying attention to proper diet and exercise, so they remain capable of taking care of patients as they age. The physician should be careful with his money to save some for old age.[24]

A later book that addresses morals was written by Abi Aly Ahmad Ibn Mohammad, known as Ibn Maskaweh. He was born in 940 CE and died in 1030 CE, almost a century after al-Ruhawi. The book is titled *Tahzib al-Akhlaq wa-tathir al-Aa'raq* (*Refinement of Morals and Purification of Lineage*).[25] Although this book is not specific to physicians, it shows the importance Islamic scholars gave to morals (ethics). Ibn Maskaweh states that if the actions of the human being are less than what he is created for by not adopting the morals outlined in Shariah, he will undermine his honored status among other creations of God. Ibn Maskaweh then discusses in detail the virtues one should acquire and the vices and bad characters one must avoid. The moral person does what he does not for worldly benefit but for God's love.

This genre of writings dedicated to morals has been called *adab* literature (Padela 2007). Contemporary *adab* literature, writings dedicated to morals pertaining to the medical profession, embraces universal virtues while expressing them with an Islamic vocabulary. An international conference on Islamic medicine held in Kuwait in 1981 synthesized a medical code from the Islamic perspective. The Kuwait Declaration consists of eleven parts. It calls for universal ideas within the framework of Islamic discourse (Padela 2007). A more recent example is Arafa's "Ethics of the Medical Profession from the Islamic Viewpoint" (Arafa 2000). It lists personal qualities considered necessary to ethical practice: sincerity, honesty, truthfulness, compassion, sympathy, patience, tolerance, and humility (Padela 2007).

The Islamic model of high moral and ethical standing was most obvious in the care provided in hospitals. The concept of a special structure, a hospital (*bimaristan*), for housing patients was first actualized in Muslim

---

24. Tahthib al-Akhlaq and Tathir al-A'araq by Aby Ahmad Ibn Mohammad Ibn Miskaweyh. Published by the Egyptian Hussainiyyah Printing company, Cairo, Egypt, 1329 H 1911 AC. Available at the American University, Cairo, Egypt (Arabic).

25. Abouleish E Contributions of Islam to Medicine J Islam Med Assn 1979; 28–45.

lands. One of the largest hospitals was al-Mansuri Hospital in Cairo, Egypt, constructed in 1284 CE. It was a place for treatment of all patients independent of wealth, social status, region of residence, creed, or race. Both men and women were taken care of, but, according to the Islamic code, they were treated in separate units. A pharmacy was part of the hospital. The hospital also had a kitchen where meals were prepared and served to the patients. Major and minor problems, including mental problems, were taken care of there. A mosque and a chapel were on the premises. The patients were kept in the hospital till full recovery. All expenses were paid by the hospital and the patients were given some money on discharge to take care for of themselves until they could start earning on their own.[26],[27]

Physician's Oath

The importance of ethics in the medical profession has been recognized from early times. The oldest known oath is the Hippocratic Oath. This and other oaths are cited in an article by Ahmad et al.[28] Hippocrates (born in 460 BC) stated in his oath "I will use my knowledge, which according to my ability and judgment, shall be for the welfare of the sick, and I will refrain from that which shall be baneful and injurious. If any shall ask me for a drug to produce death, I will not give it, nor will I suggest such counsel. In like manner, I will not give to a woman a destructive pessary (abortifacient)."

Musa Ben Maimon (Maimonides) (1135–1204 CE) has been recognized as one of the most famous Jewish theologian, philosopher, and physician. He was born in Cordoba, Spain, when it was under Muslim rule. He immigrated to Morocco, then for a short while lived in Palestine and then in Egypt, where he served as the court physician to Salah ad-Din. In addition to his several books he formulated a physician's oath and prayer. The oath reads in part:

> "Thy eternal providence has appointed me to watch over the life and health of Thy creatures. May the love for my art actuate me at all times; may neither avarice nor miserliness, nor thirst for glory or for a great reputation engage my mind; for the enemies of truth and philanthropy could easily deceive me and make me forgetful of my lofty aim of doing good to Thy children. Grant me strength, time, and opportunity always to correct what I have acquired, always to extend its domain; for knowledge is immense and the spirit of men and extent infinitely to enrich itself daily with new requirements. Today he can discover his errors of yesterday and tomorrow he may obtain in new light on what he thinks himself sure of today."

Ahmad et al note that Maimonides' oath clearly emphasizes the role of God and the humility of man before his Creator. It is obvious Maimonides's upbringing in an Islamic environment and his exposure to the writings of Islamic philosophers at the zenith of Islamic civilization had great influence on his oath.

26.   Ahmad W D, El-Kadi, Zikria B A, J Islam Med Assn 1988; 20:11–14.

27.   Maimonides's prayer.

28.   Arawi, T A The Ethics of the Muslim Physician and the Legacy of Muhammad J Islam Med assn;43:35–8.

The World Medical Association (WMA) during a meeting of its general assembly in Geneva adopted a modern version of the Hippocratic Oath.[29] This was called the Geneva Oath and was officially adopted on September 9, 1948. It reads as follows:

"Now being admitted to the profession of medicine, I solemnly pledge to consecrate my life to the service of humanity. I will give respect and gratitude to my deserving teachers. I will practice medicine with conscience and dignity. The health and life of my patient will be my first consideration. I will hold in confidence all that my patient confides in me. I will maintain the honor and the noble traditions of the medical profession. My colleagues will be as my brothers. I will not permit considerations of race, religion, nationality, party politics or social standing to intervene between my duty and my patient. I will maintain the utmost respect for human life from the time of its conception. Even under threat I will not use my knowledge contrary to the laws of humanity. These promises I make freely and upon my honor."

The wise physicians of the past realized personal behavior in private life cannot be separated from professional behavior. Islam sets the foundation for good behavior and possessing the requisite character traits to becoming a fine person and, by extension, a physician with good moral fiber, since one cannot be virtuous only in part. In other words, a physician cannot be a virtuous parent, child, or spouse yet an immoral physician. It is the entire person who is either good or not.[30]

While both older oaths recognize multiple gods in contradistinction to Islam's strict monotheism, more recent oaths such as the Geneva Oath abolish any reference to a higher deity. Also, these modern oaths eliminate any injunctions implying sexual restrictions that were included in the ancient codes. We, as Muslims, believe no oath or covenant can be binding unless it is made with God Almighty. Dr. Zikria compiled an oath from the writings of Ibn Sina, Luqman al-Hakim, and other contemporary Muslim physicians that IMANA adopted in its tenth annual meeting in 1977 as the Oath for the Muslim Physician. It begins with affirming the oneness of God, asks God to give us (physicians) the strength to be truthful and the fortitude to admit our mistakes, to make us worthy of this favored station, and to devote our lives to serve mankind whether poor or rich, Muslim or non-Muslim, black or white. I agree with the authors that it would be nice if this oath was adopted by medical schools in Muslim-majority countries in their graduation ceremonies.

"Praise be to God, the Teacher, the Unique, Majesty of the heavens, the Exalted, the Glorious, glory be to Him, the Eternal Being who created the Universe and all the creatures within, and the only Being who containeth the infinity and the eternity. We serve no other God besides thee and regard idolatry as an abominable injustice. Give us the strength to be truthful, honest, modest, merciful, and objective. Give us the fortitude to admit our mistakes, to amend our ways, and to forgive the

29. The International Islamic Code for Medical and Health Ethics Supervised by al-Awadi Abdul Rahman A, edited by El-Gindy, Ahmad Rajai. Series of Publications of Islamic Organization for Medical Sciences, Islam and Recent Medical Problems, 2005, Kuwait. Proceedings of the conference held in Cairo Egypt December 11–14, 2004.

30. Kasule O A Biomedical Ethics: An Islamic Formulation J. Isla. Med. Assn., 2010; 42:38–40.

wrongs of others. Give us the wisdom to comfort and counsel all toward peace and harmony. Give us the understanding that ours is a profession sacred that deals with your most precious gifts of life and intellect. Therefore, make us worthy of this favored station with honor, dignity, and piety so that we may devote our lives in serving mankind, poor or rich, wise or illiterate, Muslim or non-Muslim, black or white with patience and tolerance, with virtue and reverence, with knowledge and vigilance, with Thy love in our hearts and compassion for Thy servants, Thy most precious creation. Hereby we take this oath in thy name, the Creator of all the heavens and the earth and follow thy counsel as thou have revealed to Prophet Mohammad (PBUH):

"Whoever killeth a human being, not in lieu of another human being nor because of mischief on earth, it is as if he hath killed all mankind. And if he saveth a human life, he hath saved the life of all mankind."

A modern, comprehensive code of ethics for the Muslim physician was established by the Islamic Organization for Medical Sciences (IOMS) in 2004. It is divided into three parts: 1. Medical Behavior and Physician Rights and Duties. 2. International Ethical Guidelines for Biomedical Research involving Human Subjects: An Islamic Perspective. 3. Arguments of Islamic Legal Rulings on Recent Medical Issues based on the Recommendations of IOMS.[31]

Principles of Islamic Medical Ethics

Medical ethics comprises a set of moral rules and principles that guide a member of the medical profession as to how to discharge their professional responsibilities. In Western thought these rules are based on human thought and intellect with no role for religion. On the contrary, in Islamic thought these rules and morals draw their legitimacy from divine guidance as outlined in the Quran and the Sunnah. Human actions are categorized as permissible (*halal*), obligatory (*wajib*), recommended (*mandoob*), acceptable (*mubah*), impermissible (*haram*), and discouraged/disliked (*makrooh*). A vast area of *mubah* actions allows individual and collective rational and logical reasoning within universal Shariah guidelines and in fulfillment of one or more of its objectives (*maqasids*) to make judgment of what is ethical or permissible. These objectives are: preservation of religion, life (and health), intellect, progeny, and resources.

This is the process of personal reasoning (*ijtihad*), and, in the context of medicine, this is contained in medical jurisprudence (*al-fiqh al-tibbi*). Professor Kasule describes three stages of evolution of *al-fiqh al-tibbi*. During the first period (0 to circa AH 1370), it was derived directly from the Quran and the Sunnah. In the second Islamic period (AH 1370–1420), rulings on the many novel problems arising from drastic changes in medical technology were derived from secondary sources of Islamic law either transmitted by analogic reasoning (*qiyās*), scholarly consensus (*ijmā'*), or reason (*istihsan*), presumption of continuity (*istishab*), or the consideration of public interest (*istslah*). The failure of the *qiyās* to deal with many new problems led to the third stage, the modern era (AH 1420 onward), characterized by usage of the theory of purposes of the law

---

31. Beauchamp, TL and Childress JF: Principles of Bioethics 6th ed. New York: OUP, 2008.

(*maqāsid al-sharīa*) to derive robust and consistent rulings. Professor Kasule called this method independent judgment based on the purposes of the law (*ijtihad maqasidi*). This is becoming popular and will be more popular in the foreseeable future.

This theory is supplemented by five major principles of Islamic jurisprudence (*fiqh*): 1. Intention: it requires pure and sincere intention in all medical decisions and procedures. 2. Certainty: decisions are to be evidence-based and not based on subjective feelings, or at least the evidence is preponderant. 3.Injury: requires careful balancing of the benefits of an intervention versus its side effects. 4. Hardship: allows medical procedures and therapies that are normally prohibited if there is a necessity such as saving a life. 5. Custom (*urf*) or precedent: using generally accepted protocols and procedures.[32]

Modern Biomedical Ethical Problems

The significant medical and technological advances of today have raised new, challenging ethical and moral issues. In the secular West ethicists tend to depend on their individual or collective rational thinking to make moral judgments concerning these challenges. The most accepted principles used in this regard are those developed by Beauchamp and Childress: autonomy, beneficence, non-maleficence, and distributive justice.[33]

Autonomy means a patient is to make his own decisions about treatment, if he understands the different options, benefits, and risks. In effect he must give informed consent for any test, procedure, or treatment. Beneficence is doing something beneficial and preventing harm. Non-maleficence is prohibition of doing harm to others. Distributive justice requires fair distribution of benefits and burdens. This is involved in decisions to allocate healthcare resources such as personal protective equipment, intensive care beds, and ventilators in the case of pandemics such as the Covid-19, pandemic, when at the peak of its spread these were in short supply in the entire world and even in the United States.

These principles are in general agreement with Islamic principles. God commands justice, doing good, and giving to kith and kin (beneficence), and forbids all indecent deeds, evil (non-maleficence), and rebellion. God says: We have honored Adam's children.[34] Respect of the person is a major aspect of human honor and dignity. This respect gives a patient the right to make his own decisions (autonomy).

A basic purpose of Islamic law is to secure benefits for people and to protect them from harm. This is termed *beneficence* in our lexicon of today. Prophet Muhammad says, "The best of you is the one who is most beneficial to others." Kabir, one of the companions of the Prophet, narrates. "When we were with the Prophet, a scorpion bit one of us. A companion asked, 'Oh Prophet, may I do *ruqyah* (ritual supplication to heal) to him.' The Prophet replied, 'whoever can do anything beneficial to one of his brothers, he should do it.'"

---

32. The Glorious Quran Chapter 17, Verse 70.

33. Hadith No harm, no dirar.

34. Sahih Muslim. Siddiq AH, translator. Lahore: Sh.Muhammad Ashraf; 1987: 1365, hadith no. 6426.

Non-maleficence: Islamic law states that "every action that leads to harm or that prevents a benefit is forbidden. This is what is now called non-maleficence. A hadith says: no harm or reciprocating harm."[35] Even in the case of harm, Islam advises not to reciprocate harm with vengeance.

Even eating *haram* food is allowed for the purpose of protecting health and life and avoiding harm. The pertinent rule in this regard is "necessities make forbidden things permissible." The evaluation of harm is sometimes given preference over the assessment of benefits, and the potential for harm is evaluated with more stringency. Harm is seen as a grave moral failing and harmful actions are supplemented by a reminder of punishment.

Justice: Justice is an established principle in Islamic law. Allah says: "God enjoins justice and charity."[36] Justice means equity and fairness, and charity is either the acquisition of benefit or the prevention of harm. In divine tradition Prophet Muhammad (PBUH) quotes his Lord as saying, "My worshippers, I have forbidden injustice on my part and made it forbidden among you, so do not be unjust to one another."[37]

Based on the above it appears these four principles are in general in agreement with Islamic principles. In fact, Askoy (2002) states that "these principles are not something new but only one of the latest formulations of ages old common-sense principles. They are being applied in Islamic traditional and cultural societies." However, there are differences in interpretation of autonomy in particular. What should physicians do when patients refuse treatments that are critical or lifesaving? In Islam it is permissible to override this refusal as saving life is the most important goal. On the other hand, it may be possible to abide by the patient's choice even if it does not seem to be in his best interest.

Ibn Amar said that the Prophet ordered, "Do not force your sick to eat or to drink, for Allah gives them food and Allah gives them drink." This is interpreted as saying that, if a man has no desire to eat (which is his autonomous decision), then it is most improper to give him food at such a time. On the other hand, a patient who is unconscious may have to be given nutrition while respecting his autonomy, as this may be his autonomous decision if fully conscious. Also, respect for autonomy is overruled by a beneficent action in situations where public health and safety are jeopardized.

Decisions are made with consideration of their effects on a family or within a community. Individuals are often encouraged to ask and consult with members of their family or religious leaders and consider communal resources. In the context of research, women of childbearing age are often encouraged to consult with and obtain consent from their spouses and family before participating in research as subjects, given the priority of the familial unit over the individual. While refusal of care is a right conferred by current secular articulations of autonomy, the duty to protect self and avoid harm takes moral precedence for many Muslims (Rattani 2019).

Albar Chamsi notes that "For a Muslim patient, absolute autonomy is very rare; there will be a feeling of responsibility towards God, and he or she lives in social coherence, in which influences of the relatives play

---

35. Proceedings of the first International Conference on Bioethics in Human Reproduction in the Muslim World. December 10–13, 1991. The International Islamic Center for Popualation Studies & Research, Al-Azhar University, Cairo, Egypt. Editor Serour G I, 1992.

36. The Glorious Quran 68, verse 4.

37. Contemporary Medical Issues in the light of Islamic Shariah. Organized by the Society of the Islamic Medical Sciences, Amman, Jordan 1 Published by Dar al-Bashherfor publishing and distribution Vol. 1, 1995.

their roles." The patient must listen to the opinion of close family members about any treatment. The role of the family should be respected as the patients themselves agree to this role. Healthcare providers must understand that there are different cultures that do not give priority to autonomy as it is understood in the West. The healthcare provider should, under Islamic teachings, encourage the patient to avoid risky behavior and a lifestyle that would encroach on his health. He is not only a bystander providing data but a person caring for his patient or client.

Similarly, one cannot take his own life: "And do not kill yourselves." Mustafa (2014) summarizes this discussion about autonomy. "Although the underlying essence of an individual's autonomy is something which can be said to be intrinsic to the Islamic faith, the practical outward manifestations with relation to public interest, and the ultimate view of the human being's subservience to God contrast significantly with the Western philosophical model." He further states:

> A Western grounded philosophy of autonomy, which emphasizes individualism, personal gratification, and self-actualization, denies the role of faith in a supernatural being, and often also the greater importance of societal benefit and public interest over the rights of the individual. This overriding consideration can, in fact, be an example of autonomy contradicting beneficence, as a third party can be prevented from providing aid or intervention without the exclusive authority of the individual. Islam, on the other hand, does not permit man to simply behave, or indeed misbehave, as he wishes, but rather gives a holistic set of guidelines for all facets of life and an example in the life of the Prophet. This is followed by the free will to either accept or reject the divine command.

As Muslims we can reach answers based on Islamic teaching through the methods described above. There have been many attempts to resolve these questions through conferences comprising physicians, scientists, and Muslim scholars from different parts of the world and from different schools of thought. Examples of these are meetings organized by al-Azhar University, Cairo, Egypt[38]; the Society of the Islamic Medical Sciences, Amman, Jordan[39]; and the Islamic Organization of Medical Sciences (IOMS), Kuwait. The proceedings of many of these conferences have been published.

Similar conferences have been arranged in the United States by IMANA[40] and the Initiative on Islam and Medicine (Islam and Biomedicine, September 8–10, 2018[41]). The Federation of Islamic Medical Associations (FIMA) has been publishing a yearbook called the *Encyclopedia of Islamic Ethics* (2013, 2015–2019).[42] Dr. Ahmad[43] proposed a yearly conference under the auspices of the Standing Committee on Scientific and

38. IMANA-Hofstra University Ethics Symposium End of Life Issues: Ethical and Religious Perspectives Hempstead, New York, September 17–18, 2010.

39. Islam and Biomedicine, September 8–10, 2018. Organized by the Initiative on Islam and Medicine. medicineandislam.org/academics.

40. FIMA yearbook. www.fimaweb.net.

41. Ahmad WA Medical Ethics, Islamic Perspective, J.Islam Med Assn, 2005;37:64–66.

42. Athar, S. Ed. Islamic Perspectives in Medicine. A survey of Islamic Medicine: Achievements & Contemporary Issues Publisher American Trust Publications, Indianapolis, Indiana, USA, 1993.

43. Sachedina, Abdulaziz Islamic Biomedical Ethics: Principles and Application. Oxford University Press, New York, 2009.

Technological Cooperation (COMSTECH), the science and technology arm of the Organization of the Islamic Conference (OIC), to accomplish this goal.

In addition to conferences like these, several books have been recently published such as *Islamic Perspectives in Medicine*,[44] *Islamic Biomedical Ethics: Principles and Application*,[45] *Islamic Bioethics: Problems and Perspectives*,[46] and *Medical Ethics: An Islamic Perspective*.[47] Several presentations were made and papers published.[48],[49],[50],[51],[52],[53]

Discussion of these modern ethical issues is beyond the scope of this chapter, but examples of the issues include brain death, beginning and end of life, living wills, organ donation/transplantation, euthanasia, termination of pregnancy, assisted reproductive technologies, stem cell research, and cloning. This literature constitutes the second type of Islamic medical ethics literature, the first being the *adab* literature previously described.

Ethics of Clinical Research

Islam stresses the importance of the pursuit of learning through several Quranic verses and traditions of the Prophet (PBUH) to this effect. The first revealed verses of the Quran state, "Recite in the name of your Lord, Who created. He created man from a leech-like structure. Recite, and your Lord is Most Generous, Who has taught by the pen. He taught Man that what he knew not."[54]

Learning in Islam is not limited to religious studies. Early Muslim scholars used to acquire extensive knowledge not only in jurisprudence, the Quran and the Sunnah, but also in medicine, chemistry, and natural sciences. Knowledge has to be based on evidence. God says, "Can there be another God besides Allah? Say bring forth your proof if you are telling the truth."[55]

Medical progress depends on scientific research and therefore some scholars consider it a collective religious duty (*fard kifayah*). Clinical research must rest in part on experimentation on human subjects, which creates a lot of pitfalls that unfortunately led to tragedies in the past century. The most well-known are the

44. Atighetchi Dariusch MedIslamic Bioethics: Principles and Perspectives. International Library of Ethics, law, and the new medicine. Ed. David N Weisstub. Vol. 31 Springer, Dordrecht, The Netherlands.

45. Khan, M Iqbal Medical Ethics, An Islamic Perspective. Institute of Policy Studies Islamabad, Pakistan. 2013, printed by Profile Publishing.

46. Fadel, HE: Assisted Reproductive Technologies. An Islamic Perspective. Presented at Religious Values and Legal Dilemmas in Bioethics, Fordham University School of Law, New York, January 2002.

47. Fadel, HE: Developments in Stem Cell Research and Therapeutic Cloning: Islamic Ethical Positions. A Review. Bioethics. 26(3):128–135, 2012.

48. Fadel HE Ethical Aspects of prenatal diagnosis of fetal Malformations. J. Islam Med Assn 2011;43: 182–188.

49. Athar S Principles of Biomedical Ethics J. Islam Med. Assn 2011,43: 139–143.

50. Athar S advanced Directives and Living Wills for Muslims J. Islam Med. Assn 2011;43: 144–147.

51. Padela AI, Duivenbode R The ethics of organ donation, donation after circulatory determination of death, and xenotransplantation from an Islamic perspective. Xenotransplantation.2018;25(3):1–12.

52. The Glorious Quran Chapter 96, Verses 1–5.

53. The Glorious Quran Chapter 27:64.

54. Fadel H E. Ethics of Clinical Research J Islam Med assn. 2010;42:59–69.

55. WMA Declaration of Helsinki: Ethical Principles for Medical Research Involving Human Subjects. 64th WMA General Assembly, Fortaleza, Brazil, October 2013. Ferney-Voltaire, France: World Medical Association; 2013. www.wma.net/policies-post/wma-declaration-of-helsinki-ethical-principles-for-medical-research-involving-human-subjects.

Nazis' experimentation on prisoners of war, and in the United States, the non-treatment of syphilis of Afro-Americans, despite the known therapeutic benefit of penicillin, to study the natural course of the disease in a Tuskegee study. The Nuremberg Code was promulgated in 1947 as a direct result of the trial of Nazi physicians who conducted research on the prisoners of World War II without their consent. The United Nations General Assembly adopted the Universal Declaration of Human Rights in 1948 and the International Convention on Civil and Political Rights in 1966. Article seven states: "In particular, no one shall be subjected without his free consent to medical or scientific experimentation."

In parallel with these efforts, medical professionals have worked on formulating principles of the ethical use of human subjects in research. The first such document, the Declaration of Helsinki, was adopted by the WMA in 1964 in Helsinki, Finland. This was updated several times. The last was at the sixty-fourth WMA General Assembly in Fortaleza, Brazil, in October 2016. The WMA publishes a medical ethical manual that is distributed to medical journals and medical schools throughout the world. The central point of the declaration is that medical research should be subject to ethical standards that promote respect for all human beings and protect their health and rights.

In the United States, the US National Commission for the Protection of Human Subjects of Biomedical Research was created in 1974. It produced the Belmont Report in 1979, which distilled principles of ethics related to research. It addressed boundaries between medical practice and research, basic ethical principles such as respect for persons, informed consent, beneficence, justice, assessment of risks and benefits, and selection of subjects and controls.[56]

Another international organization, the Council for International Organizations of Medical Sciences (CIOMS), was founded in 1949 under the auspices of the World Health Organization (WHO) and the United Nation's Educational Scientific Cultural Organization (UNESCO). The CIOMS, in association with the WHO, undertook its work on the ethics of biomedical research in the 1970s. It produced guidelines to enable the effective application of the ethical principles set forth in the Declaration of Helsinki, particularly in developing countries. It was updated in 2002 and enumerated twenty-one guidelines.[57]

The IOMS in Kuwait evaluated this document from the Islamic perspective in a 2004 conference in Cairo. The guidelines were considered mostly in conformity with Islamic law with a few differences. A major difference is the importance Islam places on the public interest (*maslahah mursalah*). It takes precedence over private interests in special cases. It is acceptable from an Islamic point of view to use the expected significant benefits to society as a justification for risks clinical research can pose to an individual who has no possible direct diagnostic, therapeutic, or preventive benefit. This contrasts with guideline number eight of the Declaration of Helsinki. Few other differences and a more detailed discussion of all the guidelines has been previously

56. Council for International Organizations of Medical Sciences. International ethical guidelines for biomedical research involving human subjects. Geneva: CIOMS; 2002. https://cioms.ch/wp-content/uploads/2016/08/International_Ethical_Guidelines_for_Biomedical_Research_Involving_Human_Subjects.pdf.

57. Council for International Organizations of Medical Sciences. International Ethical Guidelines for Health-related Research Involving Humans, Fourth Edition. Geneva. Council for International Organizations of Medical Sciences (CIOMS); 2016. https://cioms.ch/wp-content/uploads/2017/01/WEB-CIOMS-EthicalGuidelines.pdf.

published. The CIOMS updated the guidelines, which were published in 2016. They were translated into Arabic in cooperation with the WHO's Middle East regional office and published in Cairo in 2020.

Conclusion

With the ever-expanding field of medical ethics, Muslim healthcare providers need to familiarize themselves with all the issues discussed here. We need to develop a group that specializes in the field of medical ethics. They should incorporate their scientific and clinical experience in the basic principles of Islamic jurisprudence. Religious councils should collectively engage with Muslim physicians and scientists and issue decrees (*fatwas*) about the ever-increasing medical advances. Muslim clinicians should learn about these issues to guide them in pursing research and in their clinical practice. This will prevent them from participating in unacceptable research or mistreatment of patients. They need to counsel their Muslim patients if they seek certain treatments or procedures, which may be impermissible under Islam, to ask for religious advice.

Additional References

1. Padela, AI. Islamic Medical Ethics: A primer. Bioethics 2007;21: 169–178.

2. Sohel, Z, Padela AI. An Overlooked "Inner" Dimension to an: Islamic Medical Ethics. J Islam Medical Assn of South Africa (JIMSA) 2017; 24:1–5.

3. Mustafa, Y Islam and the four principles of medical ethics. J Med Ethics 2014; 40:479–483.

4. Rattani A, Hyder AA, Developing an Islamic Research Ethics Framework J Relig Health 2019; 58:74–86.

5. Aksoy S, Elmali, A 2002. The core concepts of the four principles of bioethics as found in Islamic tradition. Medicine and Law, 21(2), 211–224.

6. Chamsi-Pasha H, Albar MA. Western and Islamic Bioethics: How Close Is the Gap? Avicenna Journal of Medicine. 2013; 3:8–14.

7. H. Arafa. Ethics of the Medical Profession from the Islamic Viewpoint. Doha, Qatar. Available at www.islamonline.net/iolenglish/dowalia/techng-2000-August-22/techng7.asp [Accessed November 20, 2006].

8. The Islamic Code of Medical Ethics. World Medical Journal 1982; 29(5): 78–80; The Kuwait Declaration: Ethics of medicine in the light of Islamic Constitution. Medical times XVI 1981; 32(6).

9. Sohel Z, Padela, An Overlooked "Inner" Dimension to an "Islamic" Medical Ethics Journal Islam Med South Africa 24 (3),2017:2–6.

10. Zamaan Sohel, Rathor YM, Abdul Rani MF, Shah ASBM, et al. The principle of autonomy as related to personal decision-making concerning health and research from an 'Islamic Viewpoint'. JIMA 2011; 43:34.

11. Abbas Rattani, Adnan A. Hyder. Developing an Islamic Research Ethics Framework J Relig Health (2019) 58:74–86.

CHAPTER 6:

Muslim Medieval Scholars' Contribution to Psychological Medicine

M. Basheer Ahmed, MD, FRCPsy, FRCP

Human psychology is the science of understanding human thinking, emotions, and behavior. Greek philosophers originally studied it as a function of the soul. From the seventh century to the fifteenth, Muslim scholars made significant contributions in every field of science and technology, as well as in the fields of psychology and psychiatry. They translated the classical Greek texts into Arabic at the excellent House of Wisdom in Baghdad in the seventh century and made many original contributions that served as the foundation of our current understanding of personality development, mental illness, and treatment.

The field of psychology was separated from philosophy in the nineteenth century when the first psychology laboratory was established in Germany in 1879 to study the mind and consciousness. In the twentieth century American psychologists focused on observable behavior as an integrated part of psychology. Later psychology became an independent discipline because of an understanding of the influences of physiology on the human mind and by eliminating abstract elements from the natural sciences.

Religion plays a vital role in human life, and famous psychologist Karl Jung emphasized its importance in attaining psychological health and mental well-being. However, the study of psychology became secularized and as a result neglected the moral and spiritual aspects of human behavior such as how to live a balanced and constructive life and finding the purpose and meaning of life. The primary focus shifted to self-satisfaction and happiness, without due consideration of the consequences of this behavior.

God reminds us every Muslim man and woman's prayer should be: *Rabbi zidni 'Ilmaa* (O Lord, increase me in knowledge (*'ilm*) (Quran 20:114). The purpose of gaining knowledge is to understand, appreciate, and unravel the mysteries of His creation. The Prophet said, "On the Day of Judgment, God will weigh the ink of the scholars and the blood of the martyrs, and the ink of the scholars will outweigh the blood of the martyrs." This demonstrates the importance Islam places on acquiring knowledge. Muslim scholars of the medieval period therefore engaged in a quest for knowledge in every field of science, technology, philosophy, psychology, and other areas.

In ancient and medieval times, people generally believed that either demonic possession or punishment from God caused mental illness. This belief led to a negative attitude toward the mentally ill and illness, particularly in Judeo-Christian and Greco-Roman societies. On the other hand, Islamic theology held a more positive position toward the mentally ill due to specific Quranic guidelines that direct special attention and protection to the mentally ill. "Do not give your property which God assigned you to manage for the insane: provide for them with it and clothe them and speak to them words of appropriate kindness" (Quran 4:5). This Quranic verse guides us about a Muslim's responsibility toward the mentally ill: those who are unfit to manage property must be treated humanely and be kept under good care by a guardian.

Islamic psychology and the knowledge of human thinking and behavior (*ilm-al nafsiat*) is the philosophical study of human thought and practice, which includes psychology, neuroscience, and psychiatry. Some Muslims believed demonic spirits and bad Jinns caused mental illness. Many medieval Muslim physicians, philosophers, and scholars believed dysfunctions of the human brain, not demonic possession, caused mental disorders. This led to the development of humane treatment for the mentally ill and establishment of hospitals for people with mental health conditions.22

Islamic Perspective on Personality Development

Sigmund Freud presented his theory of personality development in the nineteenth century, which specified that human behavior is the result of interactions among three components of the mind: 1) the id, 2) the ego, and 3) the superego. A thousand years before Freud the Quran described three inner influences on the human mind: 1) *nafs al-ammarah* or the commanding self (id); 2) *nafs al-lawwamah*, the accusatory self (superego); and 3) *nafs al-mutmainnah*, the peaceful self that guides us toward balanced behavior and peace of mind. The Quran explains how these inner forces command our psyche (mind) and tell us how to make the ultimate balance and peace of mind.

Nafs-ammarah (the passionate soul) has the domineering influence of commanding inner desires and immediate gratification. Allah says: "Indeed it is the *nafs* that overwhelmingly commands a person to do sin" (Quran 12:53) This component of our soul inclines us toward sensual pleasure, passion, self-gratification, anger, envy, greed, and conceit. The Prophet said, "Your most ardent enemy is your evil soul which resides within your body."

Nafs-lawwamah (the conscience) gives us an awareness of our imperfections and the distinction between right and wrong. Allah says: "And I do swear by the self-reproaching soul (*nafs-lawwamah*)" (Quran 75:2). This conscience is aware of evil, resists it, asks for God's grace and pardon, repents, and tries to amend behavior in the hopes of achieving salvation. The Holy Prophet said, "There are two impulses within us. One is *nafs-lawwamah*, which calls toward good and confirms the truth, and another is *ammarah*, which leads to doubt and holds untruth and encourages evil. One should seek refuge in Allah for protection."

Nafs al-mutmainnah (the soul at peace) is the highest state of spiritual and personal development where an individual attains peace and satisfaction. A satisfied soul is in a state of bliss, content and peaceful, without immoral desires. When our conscience, the *nafs al-lawwamah*, is active, we become aware that something is wrong with the way we are feeling and behaving. We can then learn to challenge negative and immoral thinking, ultimately leading us to *nafs al-mutmainnah*: "Oh reassured soul, return to your Lord well pleased, and pleasing to Him" (Quran 89:27–28).14

Freud called the concept of the *nafs-ammarah* the id and described the *nafs-lawwamah* as it is mentioned in the Quran. He elaborated further and gave a full description of the conscious and unconscious minds, then followed with a description of the id, the ego, and the superego. The id demands immediate gratification of desires and operates as a primary process, and it exists in the unconscious mind. The ego arises from the id as an intermediary between the id and the external world. The ego functions according to the reality principle, operates as a secondary process, and represents reason and common sense.

The superego (conscience) develops under the influences of parents, teachers, religion, etc. The superego develops an ever-stronger conscience against the id's inappropriate demands. The ego grows stronger and begins to exert its influence to mediate between the two powerful forces of the id and the superego.7

Describing the ego and the id, Freud gave the example of a rider of a horse named Id. The rider cannot always control the far more powerful horse, so the rider attempts to transform the will of the horse as if it is the rider's will. Amazingly, the same example was given by the fourth caliph of the Muslims, Imam Ali, long before Freud, 1,400 years ago. Is it possible that Freud was aware of Imam Ali's writing when he was describing this powerful horse, Id, and ways to control it?

Freud described the ego as an extension of the id. It attempts to satisfy the id's need for immediate gratification but resists due to the realities of the external world and the influence of the superego. This results in tension and anxiety.

The Quran emphasizes that man was given autonomy to act using the *nafs-lawwamah* (conscience), his intelligence (*aql*), and his will (*irada*) to control the *nafs-ammarah* (inner desires and immediate gratification). This control enables man to go in the direction of achieving peace within himself (*nafs-mutmainnah*).

Abu Hamid al-Ghazali, a tenth-century philosopher and theologian, described the self (personality), its ultimate purpose, and the causes of its misery and happiness. Ghazali followed Quranic verses and divided the *nafs* into the three categories described in the Quran. Al-Ghazali emphasized that the goal of the self should be to achieve the highest spiritual level of self-satisfaction and peace.

He described the concept of the self, influenced by the *qalb*, *ruh*, *nafs*, and *aql*, which all signify a spiritual entity. He stated that the self carries two qualities that distinguish man from animals, enabling man to attain spiritual perfection. These qualities are *aql* and *irada*. Intellect is the fundamental rational faculty that allows man to generalize and form concepts and gain knowledge. Al-Ghazali distinguishes between human will and animal will. Human will is conditioned by the intellect, while animal will is conditioned by instincts such as anger and physical appetite. He further writes that the heart (*qalb*) controls and rules over them and that it has six powers: appetite, anger, impulse, apprehension, intellect, and will. He states humans have all six of these traits, while animals only have three, namely appetite, anger, and impulse.

Al-Ghazali described four elements of man's nature: the sage (intellect and reason), the pig (lust and gluttony), the dog (anger), and the devil (brute character). The pig, dog, and devil rebel against the sage (intellect). He described personality as the integration of spiritual and bodily forces. Man can either rise to the level of angels with the help of knowledge or fall to the level of animals by letting his anger and lust dominate him.

He also emphasized that every person should control his/her desires (*tazkiya nafs*) or purify him/herself to develop good conduct, which can develop only from within the self.8,9

Advances in medieval Islamic psychological thought led to the development of experimental approaches to the study of the mind and the diagnosis and treatment of mental illnesses. Early Muslim scholars wrote extensively in the areas of human psychology, and most writings about the human mind are part of philosophical writings, which encompassed almost all areas of human exploration. Islamic scholars did not practice the discipline in the modern sense of psychiatry, but their work on studying the mind and proposing treatments for mental conditions was extremely important and served as a foundation for current methods of psychological treatment.

They described psychiatric treatment as treatment of the soul, mind, and heart (*al-ʿilaj al-nafs*, *al-tibb al-ruhani*, and *tibb al-qalb*). Medieval scholars frequently mentioned *tibb al-qalb* in their writings as it was a prevailing belief in the medieval period that the heart (*qalb*) was the master organ for the sophisticated cognitive and perceptive parts of the mind that has many interrelated functions. The Quran described diseases of the heart (*fiqulubihim marad*) (Quran 2:10). This is why we see *ilajul qalb* mentioned as a psychological treatment for maladaptive human behavior. The Prophet says, "Truly, in the body, there is a morsel of flesh, and when it is corrupt, the body is evil, and when it is sound, the body is sound. Truly, it is the *qalb* (heart)."18

Although psychological medicine (*al-tibb al-ruhani*) deals mainly with spiritual and mental health, medieval scholars did not completely separate spiritual medicine from physical medicine (*al-tibb al-jismani*) as the mind is regarded as an integral part of the body in Islam.10 As a result of this new understanding of mental illness, the first mental hospitals and insane asylums were built in the Islamic world as early as the eighth century. Muslims built the first mental health hospital in Baghdad in 705, in Fez in the early eighth century, in Cairo in the ninth century, and in Damascus and Aleppo in the thirteenth century.11

General hospitals in Baghdad also contained separate wards for mentally ill patients. In addition to medication for the treatment of mental illness, psychotherapy and other ancillary treatments such as baths, music, and occupational therapy were introduced, reflecting the great emphasis placed on the relationship between the illness of the mind and the body.8,15

During the golden era of Islamic civilization (seventh–fifteenth centuries), Muslim scholars discussed the concepts of psychology, psychiatry, psychotherapy, and their role in improving mental health. Abu Bakar Muhammad Zakaria al-Razi (925 CE) is a Muslim physician who introduced the methods of psychotherapy. He described in detail the symptoms and treatment of mental diseases (*al-tibb al-ruhani*) in his book entitled *Al-Mansuri*.16

It has been claimed that schizophrenia-like disorders were rarely identified before 1800 in the Western world. Based on the writings of great medieval scholars we can say that medieval Muslim physicians probably diagnosed and treated many cases of *junoon* (a severe madness like schizophrenia).22

Hundreds of Muslim scholars of the medieval period contributed to the study of psychological illnesses (*tibb-e-ruhani*, *tibb-e nafsiat*, and *tibb-e qalb*). I have selected the work of a few scholars who have made a significant contribution to the field of psychology and mental illness. Their monumental work has become the foundation for understanding the concept of personality development and recognizing and treating common minor and major mental disorders and serves as the foundation for the current knowledge of psychological medicine.

We think of sleep as a time for resting the body; however, the brain is actually quite active during sleep when dreaming. Our dreams can be soothing, mysterious, and sometimes scary. Dreams and their interpretations have been an interest of scholars. Muhammad Ibn Sirin, a seventh-century Muslim scholar, wrote a book on interpretations of dreams (*Ta'bir al-Ru'ya* and *Muntakhab al-Kalam fi Tabir al-Ahlam.*) His book is divided into twenty-five sections on dream interpretation that cover topics from the etiquette of interpreting dreams to the interpretation of reciting certain *surah*s of the Quran in a dream. He writes that it is important for a layperson to seek assistance from a Muslim scholar (alim) who could guide the interpretation of dreams with a proper understanding of the cultural context.20

Al-Kindi, an eighth-century scholar, is considered the first Muslim philosopher; he wrote over 230 books on various subjects, including sleep, dreams, eradication of sorrow, and the intellect. He also described the therapeutic value of music and was the first to experiment with music therapy. He even attempted to cure a person with quadriplegia by using music as a part of treatment.

Al-Kindi developed cognitive methods to combat depression and discussed the intellectual operations of human beings. Kindi explained sorrow as a spiritual grief (*nafsani*) caused by the loss of loved ones or personal belongings or by failure in obtaining what one seeks. He said sorrow is not within us; we bring it upon ourselves. He used cognitive strategies to combat depression and discussed the functions of the soul and intellectual operations in human beings.1,8

Al-Tabari is a ninth-century scholar who wrote about treatment of mental illness (*'al-'ilaj al-nafs*) in his book *Firdous al-Hikmah*, emphasizing the strong ties between psychology and medicine. He wrote that people with a mental health condition frequently become physically sick due to delusions, and these delusions can be treated through counseling by physicians who can win via good rapport the confidence of their patients, leading to a positive therapeutic outcome. Al-Tabari described thirteen types of mental disorders, including madness, delirium, and disorders of thought and intelligence (*fasad al-khayal wal aql*). 8,22

Muhammad Ibn Zakariya Razi (Rhazes) was one of the most well-known and respected physicians of the ninth century. Al-Razi had expertise in several medical fields, including pharmacology, pediatrics, neurology, mental health, psychosomatic medicine, and medical ethics. His books *Al-Mansuri* and *Al-Hawi* were used as textbooks in medical schools in Europe and Muslim countries until the sixteenth century. He studied the Greek medicine of Hippocrates and Galen; however, he demonstrated originality and independent thinking in his writings. He wrote books on medicine based on his observation, examination, and follow-up of patients.6,17

Al-Razi made some interesting observations about the human mind. He rejected the mind-body dichotomy of the Greek school. In his book *Tibb al-Fonoon*, he made some postulations concerning human emotional conditions and offered suggestions for their treatment. He wrote *Al-Tibb al-Ruhani*, in which he discussed ways to treat moral and psychological ailments. He wrote that sound medical practice depends on independent thinking and on treating the soul as a substance and the brain as its instrument. *Al-Mansuri* and *Al-Hawi* contained explanations for various mental illnesses and outlined symptoms, diagnosis, differential diagnoses, and treatments. He was among the first in the world to describe the concept of psychotherapy and to use it in his practice. As chief physician of the hospital in Baghdad, al-Razi was also the director of one of the first psychiatric wards in the world. He introduced psychiatric wards as a place to care for patients with mental illness. Such institutions did not exist in ninth-century Europe.17,21

According to al-Razi, mental disorders should be treated as medical conditions. After diagnosing patients with mental disorders, he treated them with medication, diet, occupational therapy, aromatherapy, baths, and music therapy. Additionally, he practiced an early form of cognitive therapy for obsessive behavior. Al-Razi described depression as a "melancholic obsessive-compulsive disorder" triggered as a result of changes in blood flow in the brain. He stated that physicians should always try to convince their patients of improvement as well as hope in the effectiveness of treatment.

Al-Razi treated his patients with respect, care, and empathy. As part of discharge planning, each patient was given a sum of money to help with immediate needs. This was the first recorded reference to the existence of a psychiatric consultation service in a general hospital and aftercare following discharge from the hospital, which was not found in Western countries until the twentieth century.

Al-Razi analyzed the different types of pleasures as sensuous and intellectual and explained their relation with each other. He wrote human needs and desires are endless and their satisfaction is impossible. We cannot accomplish anything through constant fulfillment of desires but rather through abandoning and avoiding them. He concluded that intellectual pleasure is preferable to sensual pleasure and suggested that the excellence and perfection of a man are realized only through increasing knowledge and excellent manners, and not by eating, drinking, and mating.

Al-Razi believed physicians should be modest, soft-spoken, and gentle when communicating with their patients so as to ease the anxiety of receiving unfavorable news. He stressed the importance of communicating with patients on a personal level rather than simply making them aware of their illness and using encouraging words to give patients hope of recovery; these instructions are still used today in medical education.17

Al-Razi is also known for his contributions to psychiatric ethics. He set clear standards for the professional practice of physicians. He advised physicians on how to retain the respect and confidence of their patients. At the same time, he advised patients to evaluate their physicians and demand from them a high level of integrity. He further advised patients to avoid physicians who are addicted to wine—a clear recognition of the problem of physician impairment over 1,000 years ago.6,8

Ishaq Ibn Imran, a ninth-century Tunisian Muslim physician, wrote *Maqala fil-L-Malikhuliya*, in which he addressed psychosis in melancholia (manic depressive illness). He described the diagnosis of this mental disorder, reporting its varied symptoms. The main clinical features he identified were sudden foolish acts, fears, delusions, and hallucinations, which are similar to what is described now as bipolar disorder.19

Najab ud-din Unhammad, a ninth-century physician, classified thirty different mental illnesses into nine major categories of mental disorder. The mental illnesses he described include agitated depression, neurosis, priapism, sexual impotence, melancholia, psychosis, mania, obsessive-compulsive disorders, delusional disorders, degenerative diseases, and states of abnormal excitement. He described febrile delirium (*sauda*), when patients showed impairment of memory, loss of contact with the environment, childish behavior, and psychotic agitated reaction (*junoon*), which occurs when delirium (*sauda*) reaches a chronic state. He also described nine methods of different psychological treatments.2

Al-Farabi, a great ninth-century philosopher, wrote a treatise on social psychology and stated an individual cannot achieve perfection without the aid of other individuals. It is the innate disposition of every man to join other human beings in the work he seeks to perform. Therefore, every man needs to stay in the neighborhood of others and associate with them to achieve his desired goals and community support. Al-Farabi's *Social Psychology* and *Model City* were the first treatises dealing with social psychology. His ideas contributed to the development of the concepts of community and social psychiatry.5,21

Ibn Khaldun, a fourteenth-century scholar, is considered a father of sociology who made significant contributions to the area of social psychology. His book *Muqaddimah* was a classic on the study of the social psychology of the peoples of the Arabian Peninsula, particularly the Bedouins.4

Ali Ibn Abbas al-Majusi, a ninth-century Muslim scholar, elaborated on how the physiological and psychological aspects of one patient can influence one another in his *Complete Book of the Medical Art*, where he described the anatomy, physiology, and diseases of the brain. He found a correlation between patients who were physically and mentally healthy and those who were physically and mentally unhealthy and concluded that joy and contentment could bring a better living status to many who would otherwise be sick and miserable due to unnecessary sadness, fear, worry, and anxiety. Al-Majusi advised that a person with depression (*huzn*) has to be cured as soon as it occurs because such a condition can negatively affect the human temperament and may later cause physical health problems.

Al-Majusi discussed mental illnesses in his book *Kitab al-Malaki*, where he described a type of melancholia associated with certain personality disorders. "Its victim behaves like a rooster and cries like a dog, believes that they are wolves and wanders among the tombs at night." He described this as a serious hereditary disease with fewer chances of recovery.

He also described various physical and mental disorders, including sleeping sickness, memory loss, hypochondriasis, coma, hot and cold meningitis, vertigo, epilepsy, lovesickness, and hemiplegia. He placed emphasis on preserving health through diet and natural healing rather than on medication or drugs, which he considered a last resort. He pointed out that to preserve a human's spiritual and physical health, a doctor is advised to use psychological methods of treatment notably by strengthening the spiritual and psychic powers of man—that is, by listening to good music and creating an environment that makes one happy and feel pleasant.8

Abu Zayd al-Balkhi, a tenth-century physician, wrote a book on physiology and psychiatric disorders (*Masalih al- Al bdan wa al-Anfus*), pointing out that man's construction is from both his *nafs* and his body. He argued that man's body and psychology (*nafs*) are inseparable; therefore, human existence cannot be healthy without a positive interaction between *nafs* and body. Al-Balkhi clarified the concepts of psychological medicine (*al-tibb al-ruhani, al-tibb al-qalb*) within Islamic medicine. He wrote that imbalance in the body can result in fever, headaches, and other physical illnesses, while imbalance in the soul can result in anger, anxiety, sadness, and other mental symptoms. He criticized medical doctors who concentrated only on physical illnesses and neglected psychological aspects of illnesses. Al-Balkhi said it is balance between mind and body that brings about health, and imbalance will cause sickness. One thousand years after his death we are emphasizing the cohesive function of the mind and body in medical schools.

Al-Balkhi pointed out that if an individual has a physical illness, he also suffers emotionally with loss of pleasure and interest, and depression. If a person has psychological problems, the body may develop somatic problems. Hence, the psychological condition is considered one of the main factors contributing to physical health. While supporting the idea that physical diseases should be treated through medical methods involving the use of drugs or surgery, he nevertheless encouraged psychological treatments as a part of comprehensive medical treatment. The credit goes to al-Balkhi for developing the foundation of psychosomatic medicine, which gained recognition in the West in the twentieth century.[18]

Al-Balkhi was probably the first psychologist to differentiate between neuroses and psychoses and classified neurotic disorders and to show in detail how cognitive therapies can be used to treat classified disorders. Al-Balkhi classified neuroses into four emotional disorders: fear and anxiety, anger and aggression, sadness and depression, and obsession.

He recognized two types of depression (*al-huzn*); one is caused by known reasons such as loss of loved ones, personal belongings, loss of something very valuable, or failure to obtain what one wishes to possess. This ailment can be treated psychologically through both external methods (such as persuasive talking, preaching, and advising) and internal methods (such as the development of inner thoughts and cognitions that help the patient get rid of his depressive condition).[18] This methodology is adopted now as cognitive behavior therapy (CBT), using the same principles Al-Balkhi advocated over 1,000 years ago.

The second depression is caused by unknown reasons such as a "sudden affliction of sorrow and distress, which persists all the time, preventing the afflicted person from any physical activity or from showing any happiness or enjoying any of the pleasures." which may be caused by physiological reasons (such as impurity of the blood) and can be treated by medication. This type of depression is known today as major depression caused by a depletion of the neurotransmitter serotonin, which al-Balkhi described over 1000 years ago. Al-Balkhi also introduced the concept of reciprocal inhibition (*al-ilaj bi al-did*) by describing how to reduce fear and panic (*taskin al-khawf wa al-faz'*). Reciprocal inhibition means anxiety is inhibited by a feeling or response that is not compatible with it. This concept was reintroduced over 1,000 years later by Joseph Wolpe in 1969.[8,18]

Abu 'Ali al-Husayn (Ibn Sina) (Avicenna) was a tenth-century philosopher and physician. He was born in Afshana near Bukhara. As a philosopher, he had a profound impact upon European philosophy. His major work as a physician is the *Canon* (*Al-Qanun fi'l-Tibb*). Europe and the Muslim world used this as a medical textbook until the sixteenth century. He described the diagnosis of and treatment for a variety of medical conditions, including paralysis, stroke, insomnia, vertigo, and epilepsy as well as male sexual dysfunction. He was among the earliest Muslim scholars to describe the psychiatric conditions of mania (melancholia) and depression and their treatment. He was a pioneer in the field of psychosomatic medicine, linking changes in the mental state to changes in the body. He described psychological conditions in the *Kitab al-nafs* parts of his *Kitab al-shifa* (*Book of Healing*) and *Kitab al-najat* (*Book of Deliverance*).

Ibn Sina described the concept of human self-awareness and self-consciousness independent of the perception of the body in his famous description of the floating man. If a person was created in a perfect state, but he is blind and suspended in the air, unable to perceive anything through his senses, can he affirm the existence of his self? Suspended in such a state, he cannot affirm the existence of his body because he is not empirically aware of it; thus, the argument may be seem as affirming the independence of the soul from the body, a form of dualism. In that state, he cannot doubt that his self exists because there is a subject that is thinking, confirming the self-awareness of the soul and its substantiality.3

Ibn Sina divided human perceptions into the five external classical senses of hearing, sight, smell, taste, and touch (known for a long time) and five internal senses that he described himself. Common sense collates the information gathered by the external senses. Retentive imagination remembers the information gathered by common sense. Compositive human imagination helps humans learn what to avoid and what to seek in the world around them. Estimative power is the ability to make innate judgments about the surrounding environment and determine what is dangerous and what is beneficial. For example, an innate and instinctual fear of predators would fall under this sense. Memory is responsible for remembering all the information developed by the other senses, and processing is the ability to use that information. This is the highest of the seven internal senses.12

Ibn Sina dedicated three chapters of *Canon* to neuropsychiatric disorders, in which he defined madness (*junoon*) as a mental condition in which reality is replaced by fantasy and discovered that it is a disorder of reason with its origin in the middle part of the brain. Today this condition is described as schizophrenia, which he clearly distinguished from other forms of madness such as mania, rabies, and manic-depressive psychosis. He observed that patients suffering from schizophrenia (*junoon*) show agitation, suffer behavioral and sleep disturbance, give inappropriate answers to questions, and in some cases are incapable of speaking at times. He wrote that such patients need to be restrained in order to avoid any harm they may cause to themselves or to others.

Ibn Sina also wrote about symptoms of and treatments for delirium, mania (melancholia), hallucinations, nightmares, epilepsy, paralysis, insomnia, weak memory, stroke, vertigo, and involuntary movements. He recognized the interaction between physiology and psychology in the treatment of illnesses involving emotions and developed a system for associating changes in the pulse rate with inner feelings, seen as an anticipation of Carl Jung's word association test. He postulated the theory of temperaments to encompass emotional aspects, mental capacity, moral attitudes, self-awareness, movements, and dreams. He explained that a person can overcome physical ailments through believing he can become well, and a healthy person can become physically sick if he believes he is ill, including psychosomatic illness as a part of a broad spectrum of mental illnesses.21,22

As mentioned earlier, medieval Europeans believed mental illness is caused by demonic possession. On the contrary, medieval Muslim physicians, philosophers, and scholars believed mental disorders are caused by physiological reasons affecting the brain. This led to the development of humane treatment for the mentally ill and the establishment of mental hospitals.

Muslim scholars like Razi, al-Balkhi, and Ibn Sina were the first physicians to study *al-'ilaj al-nafs*. Their works were translated into Latin, which enlightened the West and served as the foundation for current studies in psychology and psychiatry. It is amazing to see that our current knowledge of mental illness is rooted in the highly acclaimed work by medieval Muslim scholars. The world has yet to recognize this contribution.

Unfortunately, even Muslims in general are not aware of their service to global civilization. I hope this information about Muslim scholars and their heritage will serve as an inspiration to all young Muslims to follow in their footsteps.

References

1. "Al-Kindi" Stanford Encyclopedia of Philosophy, Wed Apr 11, 2018. https://plato.stanford.edu/entries/al-kindi.

2. Adamis, D.; et al. (2007), A brief review of the history of delirium as a mental disorder. https://hal.archives-ouvertes.fr/hal-00570887/document.

3. Ahmed A. "Ibn Sīnā on Floating Man Arguments." Pitzer. http://pzacad.pitzer.edu/aalwisha/pdfs/Ibn_Sina_on_Floating_Man_Arguments.pdf.

4. Akbar, A., (2002). "Ibn Khaldun's Understanding of Civilizations and the Dilemmas of Islam and the West Today, Middle East Journal 56.

5. Al-Farabi. Wikipedia. https://en.wikipedia.org/wiki/Al-Farabi.

6. Daghestani AN: al-Razi (Rhazes), 865–925. Am J Psychiatry 1997; 154:1602. https://ajp.psychiatryonline.org/doi/10.1176/ajp.154.11.1602.

7. Freud, S. (1923). The Ego and the Id. The Standard Edition of the Complete Psychological Works of Sigmund Freud, Volume XIX (1923–1925). http://icpla.edu/wp-content/uploads/2012/10/Freud-S.-The-Ego-and-The-Id.pdf.

8. Haque, A., (2004), Psychology from Islamic Perspective: Contributions of Early Muslim Scholars and Challenges to Contemporary Muslim Psychologists, Journal of Religion and Health, 43. www.jstor.org/stable/27512819?seq=1.

9. http://psychspiritual.blogspot.com/2012/03/al-ghazali-islamic-psychology.html.

10. Ibn Manzur, Lisan al-'Arab, 6 vols. (Cairo: Dar al-Ma`arif, n.d), s.v. "q-l-b," 5: 3713–3715 and "n-f-s," 6: 4500–4504; Hanna E. Kassim, A Concordance of the Quran (Berkeley: University of California Press, 1983), s.v. "n-f-s" and "q-l-b," 825–830, 903–906 respectively). http://yjhm.yale.edu/essays/ndeuraseh3.htm.

11. Ibrahim, B. S., "Islamic Medicine: 1000 Years ahead of its time." www.ishim.net/ishimj/2/01.pdf.

12. "Inner Senses." Encyclopedia. www.encyclopedia.com/humanities/encyclopedias-almanacs-transcripts-and-maps/inner-senses.

13. Jung CJ. Modern man in search of a soul. London, Routledge, 1961

14. Mahmoud, M. "The Attributes and Names of the Ranks and Stations of the Nafs in its Striving and Elevation." Basics of Islam: Types of Nafs. www.islamicity.com/forum/printer_friendly_posts. asp?TID=3949.

15. Miller, A., C. (December 2006). Jundi-Shapur, bimaristans, and the rise of academic medical centres. Journal of the Royal Society of Medicine. 99 (12). p. 615). https://archive.is/20130201153053/http:/ jrsm.rsmjournals.com/content/99/12/615.short.

16. Murad I, Gordon, H. Psychiatry and the Palestinian population. Psychiatric Bulletin (2002; 26:28). www.cambridge.org/core/journals/psychiatric-bulletin/article/ psychiatry-and-the-palestinian-population/E181752FBD63942A6DB3CD33DB89288D.

17. Musa, Y., "Muhammad Ibn Zakariya al-Razi and the First Psychiatric Ward" Sept. 2018. https://ajp. psychiatryonline.org/doi/10.1176/appi.ajp-rj.2018.130905.

18. Nurdeen, D., Mansor, Abu Talib "Mental health in Islamic medical tradition" International Medical Journal Vol. 4 No 2 Dec 2005. www.academia.edu/1273286/ Mental_health_in_Islamic_medical_tradition.

19. Omrani A., et al "Ibn Imran's 10th century Treatise on Melancholy." March 3, 2012. www.academia. edu/3885846/Ibn_Imrans_10th_century_Treatise_on_Melancholy.

20. "Psychology in medieval Islam." Wikia. https://p "Al-Kindi" Stanford Encyclopedia of Philosophy, Wed Apr 11, 2018.

21. Wael Mohamed, C.R. (2012). Arab and Muslim Contributions to Modern Neuroscience. International Brain Research Organization History of Neuroscience). http://ibro.org/wp-content/ uploads/2018/07/Arab-and-Muslim-Contributions-to-Modern-Neuroscience.pdf.

22. Youssef, H. et al. (1996), Evidence for the existence of schizophrenia in medieval Islamic society. https://journals.sagepub.com/doi/10.1177/0957154X9600702503.

23. "History of mental illness," Ancient Islam, Wikia. https://psychology.wikia.org/wiki/ History_of_mental_illness.

CHAPTER 7:

Muslim Female Physicians and Healthcare Providers in Islamic History

Marium Husain, MD, MPH,

Sharif Kaf al-Ghazal, MD, MCh(Plast.), DM, MA, Fatima Tourk, BS

Introduction

A study of the contributions of the golden age of Islamic civilization would be incomplete without enumerating the valuable contributions made by women. Although it is known that there is little information on the role of women in Islamic medical history, it is not because of the lack thereof but rather male historians' incompetence in documentation. According to some, women have not played any significant part in the development of this field. In this chapter, we will prove this assumption is not true and the role of Muslim women in the field of healthcare is wide ranging, as it is in other worldly and religious fields. We need to examine this issue in depth, and it is unfortunate that most sources relating to this are published in Arabic, which can make it difficult for non-Arabic speakers to learn about this. After extensively reviewing Islamic history and the golden age of Islamic civilization, it is very evident that women played a significant role in actively learning, practicing, and promoting medicine and healthy living from the beginning of Islam. The focus of Islamic medicine was on preserving health in times of well-being and restoring health in times of illness.

The Rise of Islamic Medicine

The practice of medicine has a special significance in Islam. The Prophet Muhammad (PBUH) instructed his companions on the importance of seeking treatment for ailments and diseases. Medical sciences gained a special interest in Islam as the Prophet (PBUH) always urged his companions to find cures using known medical treatments, which encouraged Muslims to regard the science of the human body as important as the science of religion. In fact, historians consider the tent of Rufaida al-Aslamia (Khimat Rufaida), an early Muslim woman, the first hospital on the battlefield. Historical records show that the Prophet (PBUH) himself would visit Salma um-Rafe, a freed maid of the Messenger, for the treatment of his wounds and she would apply henna.

Usamah Ibn Sharik reported: A Bedouin said, "O Messenger of God, shall we not seek treatment?" The Prophet (PBUH) said, "Yes, O servants of God, seek treatment. Verily, God did not place a disease but that he also placed its treatment or cure, except for one ailment." They said, "O Messenger of God, what is it?" The Prophet (PBUH) said, "Old age."

In another hadith, narrated by Abdullah Ibn Masud, the Messenger of God said, "One who has knowledge of it knows it, and one who is ignorant of it is ignorant." This means the Prophet (PBUH) has instructed us to seek knowledge of treatment and search for the cure of ailments. During the time of the Prophet (PBUH), there were a few female Muslim physicians who contributed to the provision of healthcare. Unfortunately, due to the dominant male bias, those who recorded history did not do justice in recording their accomplishments.

Hospitals and Home Visits

Plenty of evidence indicates women practiced in medicine from the early years of Islam. This predates Florence Nightingale's contributions to the field during the Crimean War (1853–1856). The tent of Rufaida was considered perhaps the first mobile hospital for treating patients in Islamic history, which will be explored in more detail later in this chapter. It was known that al-Zahrawi in Andalus depended on healthcare assistants who helped during his practice in obstetrics and female health (now known as midwives). In later years, it was reported that the daughter of Shehabuldin al-Saigh used to work in al-Mansouri Hospital (the biggest hospital in Egypt at the time) and held a senior position there.

Besides working in the hospitals, female physicians used to visit patients in their homes. Al-Tabari, in his book *Tareekh al rusool wa al mulook* stated that one male physician called Abo al-Hasan had one female patient come to see him with an infected wound in her shoulder and he responded by telling her, "I am a *kahal* (an eye physician) but we have a female physician who will be treating you." She saw the female physician and al-Tabari viewed this hospital (*bimaristan*) as a public health service. At the same time, there was a lot to be said about the midwives who used to visit patients in their homes. Ibn al-Hajj described this in his book (*Al-Madkhal*) when he described the life of Muslim women in Cairo during the thirteenth and fourteenth centuries and how families used to arrange for midwives to perform deliveries and look after newborns.

Specialties of Female Health Providers

The medical specialties known at the time included looking after wounded warriors and providing minor surgery as well as complicated trauma surgery such as amputation. Cauterization (*kai*) and bloodletting (*hijama*) were also practiced. Female physicians used to look after the wounds, stop the bleeding, change the dressing, and provide handmade creams to promote wound healing.

The field of obstetrics and gynecology was full of female physicians, midwives, and nurses. Their role was especially important in retaining modesty and upholding Islamic values considering the rules and regulations of Shariah.

Women were also involved in pharmaceutical creation. As mentioned earlier, in the book of al-Tabari it was stated that women helped treat infected wounds by making the right antiseptic creams. It is also well known that Zainab of Bani Oud specialized in treating eye diseases and in making topical medications. Al-Shifaa Bint Abdullah, who used to treat skin ulcers with handmade topical creams, was also appointed as the head of Husbah (the body that would regulate different businesses in the Souk, including the composition of pharmaceuticals). She was appointed by the second caliph, Omar Ibn al-Khattab.(1)

The medical profession in Muslim society was monitored by the *muhtasib*, an employee assigned to regulate and supervise all professions in the Islamic state. He was also entitled to obtain the oaths of physicians, both male and female, before they received an accredited certificate to be a professional practitioner, and to assure physicians' competence.

In his famous book *Mehnat at-Tabeeb* (*The Trial of the Physician*), Yuhanna Ibn Masawaiyh enlisted the detailed accreditation process. *Muhtasibs* recorded the fundamentals of the medical profession, the conditions of their practice, and their direct relationship with the chief physicians to whom they were assigned.

Muslim Female Physicians and Healthcare Workers

1. Rufaida al-Aslamia

Rufaida reportedly embraced Islam in the Prophet's Mosque in Medina after Hijrah and joined the Prophet (PBUH) in a few battles. She joined the army in the Battle of Badr, supporting the fighters and treating their wounds. Rufaida learned most of her medical knowledge by assisting her father, a physician named Saad al-Aslamy. In the Battle of the Trench (*al-Khandaq*), she had a medical tent (very much like the military mobile hospital used in the modern era) with all the equipment needed to treat injuries. She was the first in Islamic history to run a military mobile field medical center. She treated injured companions, as she did Saad Ibn Muaaz after the request of the Prophet (PBUH), according to hadiths, in Sahih Bukhari. She stopped the bleeding immediately and later removed the arrow from his arm in her tent.(2)

Rufaida was also allowed to put her tent in the Prophet's Mosque in Medina, where a few volunteer nurses helped her by taking shifts to look after Saad Ibn Muaaz. She trained some of the female companions in first aid and nursing before the battle of Khaybar. These female nurses ran the mobile medical military tent and took shifts around the clock to look after wounded people. That shows how the mosque during the Prophet's time was also used as a medical center. This story inspired the use of many mosques as medical, rehabilitation, and vaccination centers during the recent Covid-19 pandemic.(3,4)

The Prophet (PBUH) gave Rufaida a share of the spoils of war (*ghana'em*), similar to any fighter. She also helped treat many of the companions during peacetime. Rufaida is depicted as a kind, empathetic nurse and a good organizer. With her clinical skills, she trained other women to be nurses and to work in healthcare. She also worked as a social worker, helping solve social problems associated with disease. In addition to this, she helped children in need and took care of orphans, the disabled, and the poor.(5,6)

She trained other women to become nurses. Rufaida reported a few hadiths of the Prophet (PBUH), which were narrated by al-Bukhari, Abu Dawood, and al-Nasa'ee.(7) Many streets, schools, and places are named after her. The Royal College of Surgeons of Ireland in conjunction with the University of Bahrain grants an award named after Rufaida to distinctive students every year.(8)

2. Al-Shifaa (Laila Bint Abduallah al-Qurashiyah al-Adawiyah um-Sulaiman)

Al-Adawiyah was one of the female companions of the Prophet (PBUH) who had a strong presence in early Muslim history as she was one of the wise women of that era. She was literate in a time of illiteracy. She was the first female teacher during the time of the Prophet (PBUH). She was involved in public administration and skilled in medicine. Her real name was Laila. However, because she practiced medicine and due to her knowledge and skill, she was called al-Shifa (the healing), so her name is partly derived from her profession as a nurse and medical practitioner. Al-Adawiyah used a preventative treatment against ant bites and the Prophet (PBUH) approved of her method and requested she train other Muslim women. Because of her knowledge of reading and writing she became a teacher to Hafsah Bint al-Khattab (the Prophet's wife). She also trained her to treat skin diseases, as she was well known for treating dermatological conditions, especially eczema and skin ulcers.(12)

Al-Adawiyah was appointed by Omar Ibn al-Khattab, the second caliph, as a market inspector (*hosbah*) in Medina. She was the first Muslim woman to hold this public office, which is similar to the position of a health and safety officer in current times.(7,9)

Al-Adawiyah was the narrator of twelve hadiths of the Prophet (PBUH). She died in 641.

3. Nusaybah Bint Harith al-Ansari (um-Atiyyah al-Ansariyyah)

Nusaybah practiced medicine before and after she embraced Islam. She learned to perform circumcisions due to encouragement by the Prophet (PBUH).(9,10) Nusaybah had good relations with the Prophet's (PBUH) wives and used to visit them regularly and share gifts with them. She reportedly narrated several hadiths of the Prophet (PBUH). She joined the Prophet (PBUH) in seven battles and took care of casualties, providing the injured with water, food, and first aid.

Nusaybah washed and prepared the body of Zainab (the Prophet's [PBUH] daughter) before her burial. She is credited with narrating over forty hadiths of the Prophet (PBUH); some of them are narrated by al-Bukhari (7). One of the hadiths was about permission for women to attend Eid prayers as narrated in Sahih al-Bukhari. In her later years she moved to Basra, Iraq, where she died.

4. Nusaybah Bint Ka'ab al Maziniyyat (Om Omara)

Nusaybah was one of the early females who embraced Islam. She traveled from Medina to Mecca to meet the Prophet (PBUH) before *hijra* and was the first woman to promise the Prophet (PBUH) her support when he migrated to Medina. She was one of two women and seventy men who affirmed the agreement of Aqaba (Bay'at al-Aqabah) with Mos'ab Ibn Umair. (2) She helped the injured during the Battle of Uhud and bravely protected the Prophet (PBUH), who said that every time he looked to his right or his left he would see her fighting to defend him. During the battle she was injured in her neck.(6,9) Nusaybah kept supporting and treating the wounded after the war. During the reign of the first caliph, Abu Bakr, she continued to be a strong fighter. In the battle against Mosailimah, her arm was amputated. She returned to Medina and treated it herself.

5. Um Sinan al-Islamiyyah

Um Sinan was one of the companions who asked permission of the Prophet (PBUH) to go to the battlefield and assist the wounded and provide water to the thirsty. She joined the Prophet in the Battle of Khaybar, helping treat the wounded companions.(11)

6. Um Warqah Bint Abdullah Ibn al-Harith al-Ansariyyah

Um Warqah helped nurse the wounded. She also participated in compiling the Quran and made her house a little mosque after she obtained permission from the Prophet (PBUH) to do so. She was known to be a living martyr as the Prophet (PBUH) used to encourage his companions to go to visit the martyred woman. The Prophet (PBUH) predicted she would be killed and she was indeed killed by her own servant during the time of Umar Ibn al-Khattab.(6,12)

7. Al-Robee'e Bint Mo'awaz

Al-Robee'e lived during the time of the Prophet (PBUH). She was also one of the people who narrated a few hadiths of the Prophet (PBUH), especially the one about how he performed the *wudu*. She was one of the companions who attended Bay'at Al-Ridwan in the sixth year of Hijrah. Al-Robee'e helped treat injured companions. She died in AD 665 during the reign of Caliph Muawiya (13).

During the Prophet's (PBUH) time, more female companions helped the injured fighters in the Muslim army by providing wound dressings, splints, and herbs for pain relief. Some of them are: (1,14,15)

8. Um Hakam al-Makhzoomiyyah

9. Um Musa Ibn Nusair

10. Safiyyah Bint al-Khattab

11. Aisha (the Prophet's [PBUH] wife)

12. Um Ayman (Barakah Bint Tha'alaba)

13. Um Salim (Anas Ibn Malik's mother)

14. Umayyah Bint Qais al-Ghafariyyah

15. Layla Al-Ghafariyyah

16. Mo'azah al-Ghafariyyah

17. Um al-Ola al-Ansariyyah

18. Ko'aybah al-Aslamiah

19. Um Rafe'e (Salma). She served and looked after the Prophet (PBUH) and his household with her husband. She helped Khadijah (the Prophet's wife) during her delivery in Mecca.

20. Himnah Bint Jahash (sister of Zainab – the wife of prophet). Himnah participated in the Battle of Uhud, bringing water to the thirsty, transporting the wounded to safety, and providing necessary treatment.(13)

21. Zaynab Bint Ali. Zaynab was the granddaughter of the Prophet (PBUH). She is known for her bravery and her skills nursing wounds on the battlefield. In Iran, admirers celebrate Nurse's Day every year, commemorating her contributions. Historically, Zaynab accompanied her brother Husain to Kufah, where he challenged the Umayyad caliph and was defeated in the Battle of Karbala in 680. She was captured at the Battle of Karbala and standing before Yazid and his son Mu'awiyah, she gave such a passionate speech that he ordered her and the other prisoners to be released.

During the Umayyads' time there were a few female physicians:

22. Zainab from bani Awd, who was famous for treating eye conditions as well as surgery. Abo al-Faraj al-Asfahani mentioned her in his book (Al-Aghani); he also mentioned her in a nice poem:

أمخترمي ريب المنون ولم أزر . . . طبيب بني أود علي الأناي زينبا

23. Faridah al-Kubra moved from al-Hijaz to Syria.

24. Kharqa'a al-Amiriyyah lived and practiced in al-Hijaz.

25. Salamah al-Qiss moved from al-Hijaz to live in Syria during the Umayyads' time.

26. Hobabah lived and practiced in Basra, Iraq (she died in 723).

During the Abbasids' time a few female physicians were documented (1):

27. Motayam al-Hamishiyyah practiced in Basra in the ninth century and died in year 838.

28. Rohass lived in Baghdad and died in 859.

29. Mahbobah lived during the Abbasid caliphate (she died in 861).

30. Om Asyah (a midwife) lived in Egypt under the Toloniyah state.

31. Fadl, the freed maid of al-Mutawakkil, lived in Baghdad (she died in 867).

During the Muslims' rule in Andalus (modern Spain) a few women worked in medicine (16,17,18):

32. The sister of al-Hafid Ibn Zohr (the grandson of Ibn Zohr [Avenzoar]) and his two daughters practiced obstetrics and midwifery as well as treating sick children (both of them were the private physicians of the wife of the ruler, al-Mansoor, in al-Andalus). There were a few physicians in the family of Ibn Zohr over five generations in al-Andalus (Ishbilya – Seville).

33. The daughters of al-Zahrawi were known to practice medicine after being taught by their father. Al-Zahrawi wrote a medical encyclopedia called *Al-Tasrif* (19) and he allocated ten chapters to discuss midwifery and obstetrics in great detail in the thirtieth volume, which was about surgery.

34. Om al-Hasan Bint al-Qadi al-Tanjaly lived in al-Andalus in the fourteenth century and was famous for practicing and teaching medicine. She was not keen on writing books, as she mentioned in her poem. She was also a scholar and taught Tajweed the Quran.

In Damascus (Syria) there was:

35. Bint Dohn al-Louz was a very skillful woman practicing medicine, who was also one of the Islamic scholars in Damascus. She died in 1216.(9)

In Egypt in the seventeenth century there were:

36. Bint Shihab al-Deen Ibn al-Sa'egh practiced medicine after she took over after her father died in 1627. She became the chief physician in al-Mansouri Hospital in Cairo (Egypt) (9). The function of that position included regulating the medical body in the biggest hospital in the country at that time.

37. Um Ahmad practiced as a midwife during the Mamluk era in Egypt.

38. The freed maid of Abi Abdullah a-Keenan practiced in al-Maghreb.

Women surgeons in fifteenth-century Turkey:

Between those first names of early Islamic history, other women practiced medicine and nursing. Few of them were recorded. However, a serious investigation in the books of the history of medicine and writings from the time will certainly provide precise data about their lives and achievements. In the fifteenth century, a Turkish surgeon, Serefeddin Sabuncuoglu (1385–1468), author of the famous manual of surgery *Cerrahiyyetu'l-Haniyye*, did not hesitate to illustrate the details of obstetric and gynecological procedures or to depict women treating and performing procedures on female patients. He also worked with female surgeons, while his male colleagues in the West reported against the female healers.

Female surgeons in Anatolia generally performed gynecological procedures like surgical managements of fleshy growth of the clitoris in the female genitalia, imperforated female pudenda, warts and red pustules arising in the female pudenda, perforations and eruptions of the uterus, abnormal labor, and extraction of an abnormal fetus or placenta. Interestingly, in the *Cerrahiyyetu'l-Haniyye*, we find illustrations in the forms of miniatures indicating female surgeons. It can therefore be speculated that they reflect early (fifteenth century) female surgeons treating pediatric neurosurgical diseases like fetal hydrocephalus and macrocephalus.(20)

The attitude toward women in the history of medicine reflects the general view that society held of women during the period. It is interesting that in the treatise of Serefeddin Sabuncuoglu, we find an open-minded view of women, including female practitioners in the complex field of surgery.(20)

39. Fatima al-Fihriyya of Morocco played a great role in the civilization and culture of her community. She migrated with her father, Mohamed al-Fihri, from Qayrawan, Tunisia, and traveled to Fez. She grew up with her sister in an educated family and learned *fiqhs* and hadiths. Fatima inherited a considerable amount of money from her father, which she used to build a mosque for her community. Established in the year 859 CE, the Qarawiyyin mosque later functioned as a university and was considered the oldest, possibly the first, university in the world (21). Students traveled from all over the world to study there.

Conclusion

Muslim female healthcare providers during the early stage of history, who participated in different aspects of medicine, are unfortunately underreported. Ibn Abi Usaibi'aa mentioned only one female physician in his book. Muslim women have had a great impact in the scientific field and more research is needed to understand their contributions. A reason for the lack of reporting of their work is that little was written about them, and that which has been written is mainly in Arabic. Unlike their male counterparts, they did not write books or articles. Interestingly, one of the well-respected female Muslim physicians, Om al-Hasan Bint al-Qadi al-Tanjaly, who lived in al-Andalus, was not keen on writing about her experience in books and she mentioned a poem in Arabic that made reference to the fact that "writers write and doers do."

الخط ليس له في العلم فائدة . . . وإنما هو تزيين بقرطاس

والدرس سؤلي لا أبغي به بدلاً . . . بقدر علم الفتى يسمو على الناس

Hence, she was so busy working she would have no time to write! It is worth remembering that the first registered female physician in England was Elizabeth Blackwell in 1858. She came from the United States, where she had qualified in 1849. It is therefore clear that there is a rich history of female Muslim physicians and healthcare workers in Islam that goes back centuries. Much can be learned from their findings, but more scholarship is needed to understand and appreciate their contributions.

References

1. Al-Nisa'a Wa Mihnat Al-Tib Fi Al-Mojtama'at Al-Islamiyyah, by Omaymah Abu Bakr & Huda Al-Sa'di, Cairo (Egypt) 1999.

2. Omar Kasule, "Historical Roots of the Nursing Profession in Islam." www.nursingworldnigeria. com/2015/02/historical-roots-of-the-nursing-profession-in-islam (accessed on December 15, 2020).

3. Muslim scholars are giving *fatwa* towards allowing mosques to be used for Covid patients' rehabilitation. https://mubasher.aljazeera.net/news/politics/2020/4/11/%D8%B9%D9%84%D9%85%D8%A7%D8%A1-%D8%A7%D9%84%D9%85%D8%B3%D9%84%D9%85%D9%8A%D9%86-%D9%8A%D8%B5%D8%AF%D8%B1-%D9%81%D8%AA%D9%88%D9%89-%D8%A8%D8%B9%D9%84%D8%A7%D8%AC-%D9%85%D8%B5%D8%A7%D8%A8%D9%8A (accessed on January 25, 2021).

4. Birmingham Mosque becomes UK's first to offer Covid vaccine. www.bbc.co.uk/news/uk-england-birmingham-55752056 (accessed on January 25, 2021).

5. R. Jan, "Rufaida Al-Asalmiy, The first Muslim nurse." Journal of Nursing Scholarship, 1996 28(3), 267–268.

6. Great women in Islamic History: A forgotten legacy. https://funci.org/great-women-in-islamic-history-a-forgotten-legacy/?lang=en (accessed on December 21, 2020).

7. The Top Hundred Female Companions during the Prophet's Time. By Mahmoud T Halabi (published in Beirut, Lebanon, 2004). (in Arabic).

8. https://en.m.wikipedia.org/wiki/Rufaida_Al-Aslamia (accessed on December 21, 2020).

9. Al-Tib wa Ra'idatoho al-Muslimat, by Abdallah al-Sa'eed, published in Amman, Jordon, 1985 (in Arabic).

10. Abdel-Hamid 'Abd Rahman al-Sahibani, Suwar min Siyar al-Sahābiyāt, Riyadh: Dar Ibn Khazima, 1414 H, p. 211; 'Umar Kahala, A'lam al-nisa', Damascus, 1959, vol. 5, p. 171.

11. www.sahaba.rasoolona.com/Sahaby/26756/ت‌ص‌ف‌ح‌-م‌ف‌ص‌ل‌/أم‌-س‌ن‌ان‌-الأس‌ل‌م‌ي‌ة (accessed January 20, 2021).

12. Great women of Islam, by Ghandafar (translated by J M Qawi). hwww.islamicstudies.info/history/companions/Great_Women_of_Islam.pdf (accessed December 21, 2020).

13. On the Position of Women in Islam and in Islamic Society (www.peacepalacelibrary.nl/ebooks/files/turabi.pdf (accessed December 15, 2020).

14. Sahabiyat Hawla al-Rasoul, by Mahmoud al-Masri (Egypt, 2005) (in Arabic).

15. The top hundred female companions during the prophet's time. By Mahmoud T Halabi (published in Beirut, Lebanon, 2004) (in Arabic).

16. Aalam al-Nisa'a fi Alamai al-arab wal Islam, by Omar Rida Kahalaih (part 1, page 259) (in Arabic).

17. The History of Medicine and Its Ethics, by Ahmad Shawkat al-Shatti (Damascus, 1960) (in Arabic).

18. Uyun al-Anba'a fi tabaqat al-Atibba'a, Ibn Abi Usaiba'a, thirteenth century (in Arabic).

19. Al-Zahrawi. Manuscript of al-Tasrif copied by Abu al-Hasanat Qutb al-Din Ahmad (year 1908). https://dl.wdl.org/7478/service/7478.pdf (accessed on July 7, 2020).

20. https://muslimheritage.com/womens-contribution-to-classical-islamic-civilisation-science-medicine-and-politics (accessed on July 7, 2020).

21. https://whc.unesco.org/en/list/170/#:~:text=Video,Medina%20of%20Fez,the%20capital%20of%20the%20kingdom (accessed on December 2, 2020).

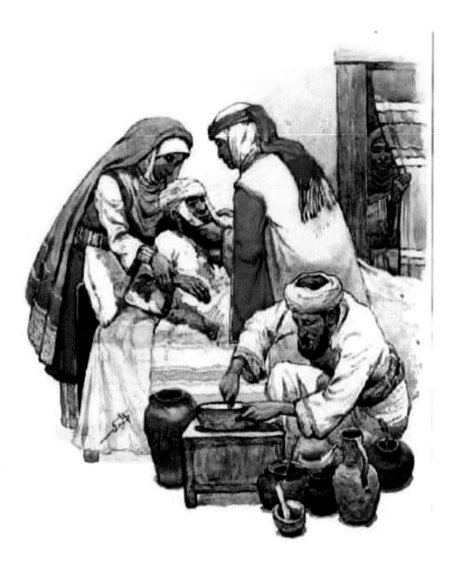

Muslim women actively participated in helping the injured during battles.

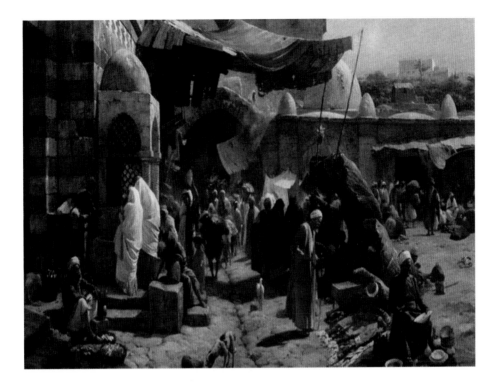

Al-Shifaa was one of the first women in Islam participating in al-Husbah (regulating and monitoring the market)

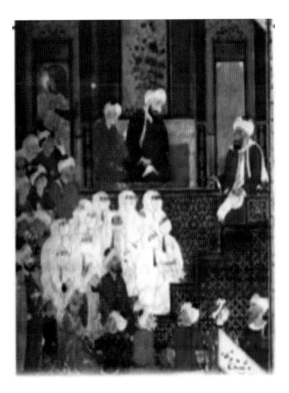

Muslim women attending a lecture and sitting in the first row

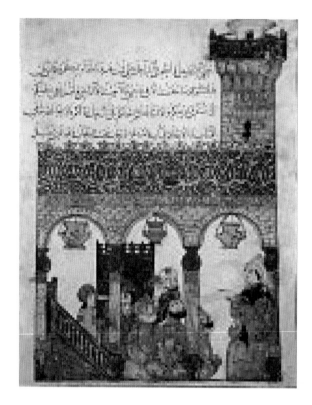

A Muslim woman teaching a group of men inside a mosque

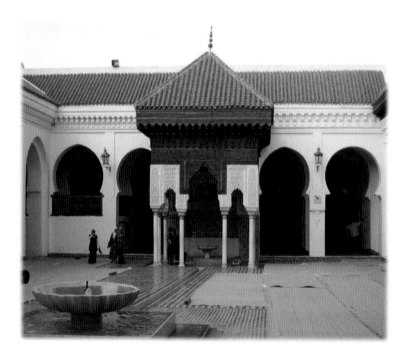

Fatima al-Fahriyya established the first university in the world,
Qarawiyyin University in Fez (Morocco) in 859 AD

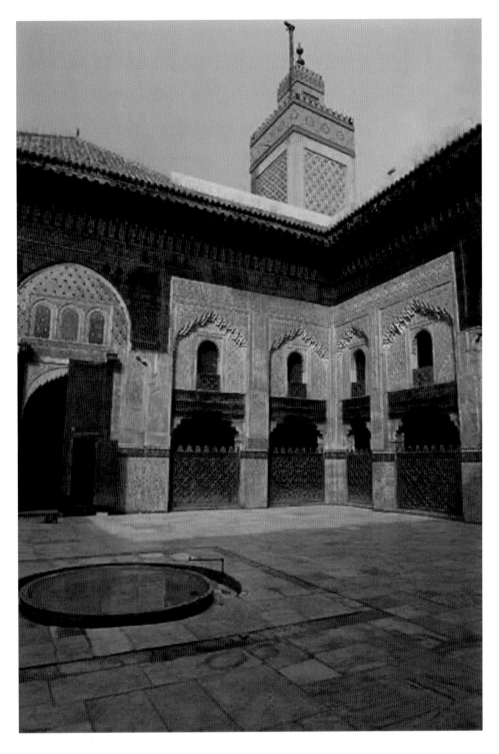

Another view of the Qarawiyyin University established in 859 CE

CHAPTER 8:

Modern Muslim Heroes of Medicine

Mubin Syed, MD, Feras Deek, MS, Azim Shaikh, MD, MBA, Mahmood Hai, MD, FICS

In this chapter, we uncover a remarkable and relatively unknown narrative - the continued contributions of contemporary Muslim doctors and biomedical researchers to the field of medicine. While the golden age of Islamic medicine, which shone brightly a thousand years ago, is widely celebrated, it is time to shift our focus to the present and shed light on the transformative innovations occurring today. These modern Muslim innovators have emerged as unsung heroes, often surpassing the achievements of their esteemed predecessors and revolutionizing critical domains such as neurosurgery, ophthalmology, cardiology, oncology, endovascular surgery, urology, and cardiac surgery. Surprisingly, their recognition and appreciation predominantly come from non-Muslims, as the Muslim community often overlooks their immense importance. However, through their inspiring stories, we have an opportunity to inspire pride and cultivate future role models for our Muslim youth, especially given the challenging climate of Islamophobia. Join us now as we embark on a journey to discover a "modern age" of Islamic medicine, where groundbreaking advancements shape the trajectory of healthcare and push the boundaries of human potential. One could claim that the golden age of Islamic medicine—dating back 1,000 years—never went away but is here and now.

We acknowledge that this list may not include all the great modern Muslim contributors to medicine, as many logistical aspects factored into their inclusion. One limitation is the lack of awareness of their contributions and the ability to contact them and obtain their consent for inclusion, as well as numerous honorees who unfortunately declined to be included. We humbly apologize to the many modern Muslim physicians and scientists in the field of medicine who have substantially enhanced their fields of practice and who were not included in this compilation. Importantly, observance of Islam in daily life was not a criterion for inclusion in this list.

Shahbuddin Rahimtoola

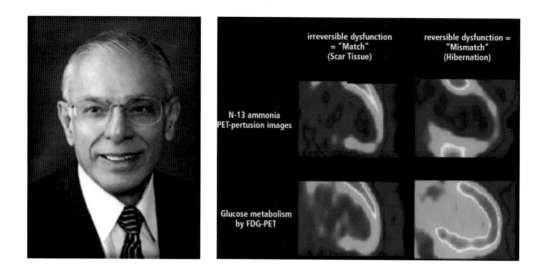

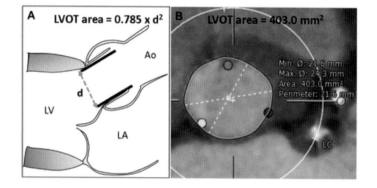

Figure Caption 1: Illustration of a "sleeping heart" demonstrating inactive/hibernating myocardium.
Figure Caption 2: Diagnostic imaging of a prostheses that is mismatched to a patient's anatomy.

DOB & Place: October 1931, Pune, India
Death & Location: December 9, 2018, Los Angeles, California

Do the terms hibernating myocardium or patient-prosthesis mismatch sound familiar? These are some of the most important concepts in modern cardiology. Hibernating myocardium refers to a part of the heart muscle that is alive but not functioning optimally due to insufficient blood flow. The main idea behind hibernating myocardium is that, once blood flow is restored, the heart muscle can recover and function normally again. This concept becomes critical as it can be the determining factor between life and death by restoring the heart's functionality in that specific area. Re-perfusion of hibernating myocardium, where blood flow is reintroduced, can significantly enhance survival chances when medications prove ineffective and the prognosis is otherwise grim.

Dr. Shahbuddin Rahimtoola was the first to describe the phenomena of hibernating myocardium. This paved the way for effective and directed coronary artery bypass graft surgery and coronary artery stenting. As of 2019 there are nearly 4,000 references in the peer-reviewed medical literature relating to hibernating myocardium.

Dr. Rahimtoola is also noted for realizing that valve surgery often failed because the size of the valve was too small for the patient. He coined the term prosthesis-patient mismatch and derived the specific criteria for grading the degree of severity. This mismatch is present in nearly 20–70 percent of artificial valve prostheses implanted every year. It has been reported that patients with prosthetic mismatch after aortic valve replacement had worse functional class and exercise capacity, reduced regression of left ventricular (LV) hypertrophy (i.e., enlargement), inferior recovery of coronary artery flow reserve, impaired blood coagulation (i.e., clotting) status, and more adverse cardiac events after surgery compared with patients without a mismatch. Of note, the term coronary arteries mentioned above are the blood vessels that feed blood to the heart. Dr. Rahimtoola was one of the first to outline the issue of prosthesis-patient mismatch, as well as the clinical complications that accompanied this mismatch.

His sobriquets were "cardiologist of the world" and "father of research," and he is listed as a contemporary giant. Many references citing him include dedications written to him. He is considered one of the top fifty all-time practitioners from the prestigious Mayo Clinic.

Ayub Ommaya

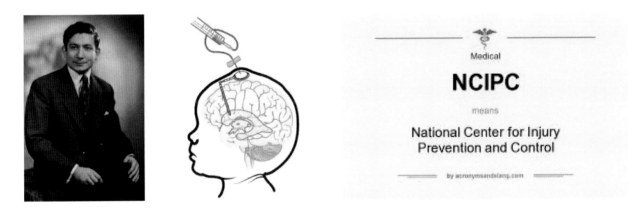

Caption: Figure 1: Illustration depicting an implanted Ommaya Reservoir for the delivery of therapies.

DOB & Place: April 14, 1930, Mian Chanu, Punjab, Pakistan
Death & Location: July 11, 2008, Islamabad, Pakistan

Traumatic brain injury has gained great notoriety in recent years, particularly due to its prevalence in major sports such as football and boxing. Traumatic brain injuries were relatively misunderstood, therefore, effective methods of studying and modeling them were virtually nonexistent until the early twentieth century.

Everyone is probably familiar with the huge controversies in today's public discourse about concussions and identifying them.

Traumatic brain injuries affect one and a half million Americans and up to seventy million people worldwide per year. Dr. Ayub Ommaya was the first to do research/modeling in traumatic brain injuries and classify them in the American healthcare system. Originally intending to study consciousness, Dr. Ommaya was led by his inquisitive mind to focus on describing, classifying, and modeling the types and biomechanics of traumatic brain injuries as well as their clinical impacts.

He is credited with starting the Centers for Disease Control's (CDC) National Center for Injury Prevention and Control via his 1985 report "Injury in America." His impact in shaping public policy and research in traumatic brain injuries and health overall truly cannot be understated.

He was a neurosurgeon by training but went on to establish critical techniques and methods in many fields within and outside his original training in medicine.

He was a prolific physician-scientist inventing a type of implantable reservoir called the Ommaya Reservoir. The Ommaya Reservoir eliminated the need for patient's frequent painful lumbar punctures to monitor or treat cancers in the brain. This invention permitted such procedures to be performed without the agony associated with lumbar punctures during the time.

On a personal note, Dr. Ommaya had two children who struggled with Type 1 diabetes. Motivated by his personal experience with the disease, he focused on the problem of transplantation of islet cells to treat it. He even developed the concept of creating an artificial organ that would house transplanted islets cells and was successfully tested in animals.

He classified nontraumatic rhinorrhea as resulting from high pressure leaks and normal leaks, thus producing seminal work in the field. Additionally, he made critical contributions to the development of spinal angiography and interventional neuroradiology. He coauthored one of the first treatments of spinal-arterio-venous malformation using steel pellets. Interestingly, known as the singing neurosurgeon; he was, in fact, an operatic tenor. Dr. Ommaya has received numerous accolades and accomplishments and is very much a giant in terms of his contributions.

Abdul Aziz

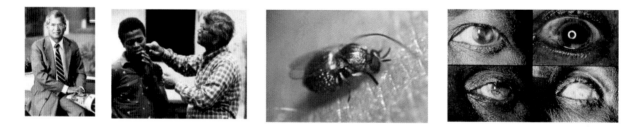

Figure 1: Picture of the fly that carries and infects humans with onchocerciasis.
Figure 2: Image depicting the effects of River Blindness on the eye.

DOB & Place: 1930, Bangladesh

Death & Location: November 25, 1987

Imagine a disease that doesn't necessarily kill you but causes blindness, leaves you so miserable as to cause severe itching to the point of self-mutilation, renders you unable to sleep or concentrate, forces you to become a social outcast due to the various dramatic ailments it produces, and even drives its victim to suicide. River blindness plagued most of Africa and parts of Latin America for most of the twentieth century, affecting countless millions. It is spread by the bite of the female black fly (genus: simulium) that hosts an infectious parasitic nematode worm (onchocerca volvulus). This infection is endemic to many parts of Latin America and Africa and was a scourge throughout the world. Dr. Mohammed Abdul Aziz was the main figure behind providing and distributing one of the most effective cures for river blindness (ivermectin), which has been used in over a billion cases of river blindness. Ivermectin has gained notoriety as it has recently wrongfully been used to treat COVID-19. Nearly 100 million people a year are treated with a preventive dose, which is responsible for eradicating the disease in many areas of Africa and Latin America.

Dr. Aziz was also instrumental in the effort to make this drug free to communities that could not afford it. Sadly, he passed before full recognition of his fantastic accomplishments was possible. Had Dr. Aziz not passed away early in his career, he would have almost assuredly received the Nobel Prize for his outstanding accomplishments. His work did, however, directly lead to the Nobel Prize in Medicine in 2015, which was instead awarded to his junior colleague William C. Campbell.

The Nobel Prize Committee specifically credited Dr. Aziz in the following statement: "In 1981 1982 Dr. Mohammed Aziz at MDRL, an expert in River Blindness, conducted the first successful human trial (Aziz et al. 1982). The results were clear. Patients given a single dose of ivermectin showed either complete elimination or near elimination of microfilariae load, while the adult parasites were untouched."

Sherif Zaki

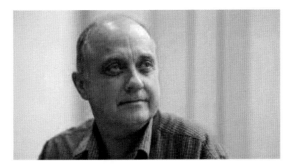

DOB & Place: November 24, 1955, Alexandria Egypt

Death & Location: Atlanta, GA, November 21, 2021

Infectious diseases are one of the major killers of mankind. Many diseases have been featured in the news. You may have heard of outbreaks of Ebola in West Africa, a disease that has a mortality rate of up to 90 percent.

How about the Zika virus, which ravaged Brazil recently and was found in the brains of miscarried fetuses? Or anthrax, which was used to terrorize members of the US government in 2001?

Dr. Sherif Zaki, a legendary disease detective and chief of the CDC's infectious diseases pathology branch, was historically significant to CDC-led epidemiologic and laboratory investigations. His contributions in diagnosing unexplained illnesses and outbreaks played a critical role in saving lives. The current director of the CDC, Rochelle Walensky, described Dr. Zaki as critical in diagnosing unexplained illness and outbreaks that allowed the CDC and public health officials to respond more quickly and save lives. Dr. Zaki headed the agency's Unexplained Deaths Project, an elite team responsible for figuring out the causes of mysterious deaths in the United States every year. He used the latest tools of modern medicine called immunohistochemistry to solve these unusual and new outbreaks of disease.

Four people who received organ transplants from a single person in Massachusetts and Rhode Island died. Dr. Zaki and his team found they all died from a rare virus carried by rodents called lymphocytic choriomeningitis. The origin was mysterious until the team discovered the organ donor's daughter had a pet hamster.

In 2005 Dr. Zaki was consulted about a boy who had fever, headache, and itch scalp. The boy had become so agitated he bit one of his relatives. Dr. Zaki diagnosed the child, who died two weeks later, with rabies. It was later discovered that the boy had dead bats in the home and that he had found a live bat in his bedroom. These difficult cases and many others, including Covid-19, West Nile Hantavirus, and severe acute respiratory syndrome, were cracked or solved by this "legendary disease detective" who was the chief of the CDC's infectious diseases pathology branch. Sherif Zaki was considered among the most influential infectious disease pathologists of his generation. In 2022 the CDC posthumously honored him with a special tribute titled "We Were There" because he was historically important to CDC-led epidemiologic and laboratory investigations.

Salim Yusuf

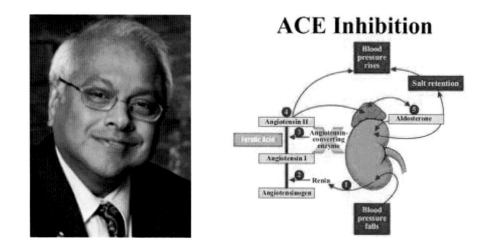

Figure 1; Graphic depicting hormonal influences on the kidney that could be disrupted to lower blood pressure through ACE inhibitors.

DOB & Place: November 26,1952, Kottarakara, India

Residence: Hamilton, Ontario

Did you know a class of drugs called angiotensin-converting enzyme (ACE) inhibitors are one of the most fundamental and widely used drugs for the treatment of high blood pressure and heart failure? Cardiovascular diseases are the leading cause of death throughout the world. Given the severity and devastation they produce, discovering ways to limit the disease are of utmost importance. By inhibiting an unregulated hormonal system, ACE inhibitors help dilate blood vessels without increasing the workload of heart. In a 2014 study ACE inhibitors were shown to produce a 10 percent reduction in relative risk for all-cause mortality and a 12 percent reduction in cardiovascular mortality, thus highlighting their life-saving impact in healthcare.

Dr. Salim Yusuf, a cardiologist born in Kerala, India, was the leading voice and researcher of the many possible benefits ACE inhibitors and beta-blockers provide for heart health. His epidemiological studies were groundbreaking in terms of their power, size, and scope, and highlighted his steadfast, determined work ethic as a prolific research physician. Dr. Yusuf had many other major accomplishments in elucidating the risks of heart diseases and the benefits of treatment. The first was showing conclusively the benefits of using aspirin and thrombolytics in heart attacks. According to Google Scholar, his works have been cited over 320,000 times! As well as identifying the risk factors for 90 percent of strokes and heart attacks, Dr. Yusuf's extensive works and impact perfectly demonstrate his passion for bringing awareness and reducing the world's burden of this number 1 killer, making realistic his life goal to reduce the burden of heart diseases globally by 50 percent in a generation.

Did you know the standard by which modern medical knowledge advances is through large international clinical trials? We now take these efforts for granted in the field of epidemiology (i.e., the study of disease patterns). Dr. Salim Yusuf has provided modern medicine with the enduring gift of the methodology of conducting large-scale international clinical trials to prove simple concepts using a collaborative network of researchers throughout the globe. His contribution to medical science has helped establish a much deeper understanding of the key principles that underlie epidemiological research. This work has led to major advances in our understanding of cardiovascular and cerebrovascular disease. He has published more than 800 articles in peer-reviewed journals, rising to the second-most cited researcher in the world for 2011. He is also the president-elect of the World Heart Federation, where he is initiating an emerging leaders program in 100 countries.

Amman Bolia

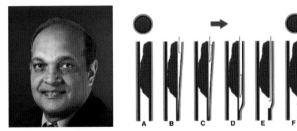 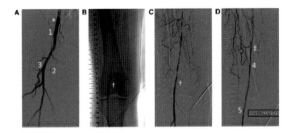

Figure 1: Steps involved in subintimal angioplasty to cross a difficult lengthy occlusion.

Figure 2: Diagnostic imaging demonstrating the treatment of a chronic total occlusion.

DOB & Place: January 8, 1953, Kigezi, Uganda
Residence: Leicester, UK

Peripheral (outside of the heart) vascular disease, or the narrowing or occlusion of blood vessels in the extremities, affects nearly eight million Americans per year and one hundred and eighteen million people worldwide. One form of effective nonsurgical treatment is percutaneous intervention. Nonsurgical endovascular treatment of arterial occlusions has become the standard of care not only for vascular interventionists but also for vascular surgeons. One of the most difficult things to treat percutaneously in peripheral arterial disease is a chronic total occlusion—especially if it is long, which happens in about forty percent of cases. Typically patients with this condition are referred for surgery, and it is a very challenging presentation to treat. You cannot really get through such hard occlusions with ease and safety to open clogged vessels. Lack of treatment for chronic total occlusions may lead to bypass surgery or amputation.

However, Dr. Amman Bolia, an interventional radiologist based in the United Kingdom, devised a technique that would revolutionize the treatment of chronic total occlusions during peripheral vascular interventions. His subintimal angioplasty procedure allows physicians to create a new pathway safely, quickly and inexpensively accessing a vessel's subintimal space to tunnel past an occlusion and provide critical treatment where it was not previously possible.

Sadly, when Dr. Bolia first presented his technique at an international vascular meeting, it was dismissed by esteemed leaders in endovascular intervention as extreme and on the fringe at that time and for many decades after. One major thought leader at that meeting warned "this experimental technique has no basis, and could be dangerous, and any dissection during an angioplasty procedure is really a complications, and cannot be allowed to be done intentionally".

Since then, his technique has become mainstream and de rigueur in the armamentarium of any endovascular specialist. Dr. Bolia has received international recognition for this major and fundamental breakthrough in preventing amputations. "I believe in medicine that works simply and efficiently and is readily available to both the practitioner and the patient," he said. "And I'm driven to find medical techniques and devices that make this possible."

Aziz Sançar

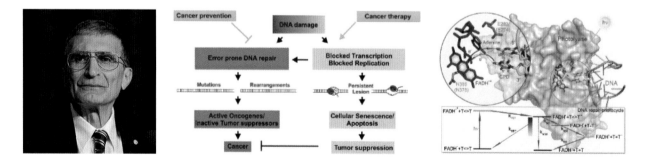

Figure 1: Graphic demonstrating the mechanism of DNA-targeted cancer treatments.
Figure 2: Illustration of the photolyase enzyme.

DOB & Place: September 8, 1946, Savur, Turkey

Residence: Chapel Hill, North Carolina

Do you know who won the Nobel Prize in Chemistry in 2015? The processes involved in DNA replication and repair constitute some of the most fascinating and intricate areas of scientific research. Understanding the underlying mechanisms could lead to great leaps in the treatment of many ailments such as cancer. Dr. Aziz Sançar received the Nobel Prize in Chemistry for his description of DNA-repair mechanisms that are found in every living organism. Dr. Sançar came from a rural family and worked as a farmer and goat herder as a young boy. He went on to study biochemical mechanisms and studied the DNA enzyme photolyase, a molecule that repairs DNA damage caused by ultraviolet light. Dr. Sançar and his colleagues earned the Nobel Prize for their work in elucidating nucleotide excision repair (i.e., a type of DNA repair mechanism); which upended this entire field of research.

Dr. Sançar has made groundbreaking contributions to the study of circadian rhythms - the natural clocks within our bodies that synchronize with the Earth's rotation, distinguishing night from day. His pivotal research delved into the genetic encoding of these clocks, offering potential insights into treating various disorders linked to disrupted circadian rhythms.

Dr. Sançar, originally a primary care physician, graduated from medical school and initially practiced in Turkey. Despite being a physician by training, Dr. Sançar's true passion lay in scientific research. Consequently, he immigrated to the United States with the aim of applying for a Ph.D. program in research at the University of Texas in Dallas, recognizing the country's abundant opportunities and resources for advancing his scientific pursuits. However, because of his thick accent, he could not get a postdoctoral position at any of his desired labs. Instead, he took on the role of a technician to persist in researching his area of interest. Surprisingly, even with a Ph.D., the only available job he could secure was that of a technician! He eventually worked his way up to do such fundamental work in advancing his field of biochemistry, that he received the prestigious Nobel Prize for Chemistry in 2015.

Tofigh Mussivand

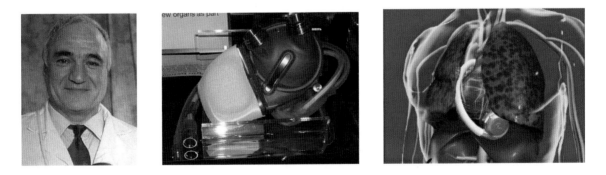

Figure 1; Artificial cardiac pump.
Figure 2: Illustration of an implanted artificial cardiac pump.

DOB & Place: 1936, Varkaneh, Iran

Residence: Ottawa, Canada

Does anyone know when the artificial cardiac pump was invented? Left ventricular heart failure affects nearly six million Americans yearly and up to twenty-six million worldwide. Due to the nature of the condition and the treatments available, the only possible option to those with severe heart failure was to wait on a donor list for a heart transplant. What if there was a machine that could do the task of pumping blood to the body?

Ventricular assist devices (cardiac pumps) did the heart's work for it, delivering blood to the body when the heart could no longer do so. The first working artificial cardiac pump was invented by Dr. Tofigh Mussivand in 1993, who, like medical pioneer Dr. Aziz Sançar, was a goat herder during his youth. This device could be completely implanted inside the human body. He surprised his colleagues by developing this device within four years. Dr. Mussivand was even able to figure out how to transfer power to recharge the device through the skin.

Dr. Mussivand has received numerous awards and was named Innovator of the Year. He was once recognized as one of the seven brightest people in the world by an American program but declined to participate.

Apart from the artificial heart used to treat heart failure, Dr. Mussivand has made groundbreaking contributions in various fields, such as advancing remote power transfer for implantable medical devices, enabling remote patient monitoring through telemedicine, studying biofluid dynamics to minimize thrombosis in blood-conducting devices, and developing technology capable of tracing a person's DNA from their fingerprint. A prolific author of over 250 papers, books, and technical articles, Dr. Mussivand has mentored over 300 postdoctoral fellows. He is an editor for many international medical journals and research institutions in the United States and Canada. Over the last decade, Dr. Mussivand's innovations have attracted investments totaling around $600 million to the Canadian economy.

Muhammad Basharat Yunus

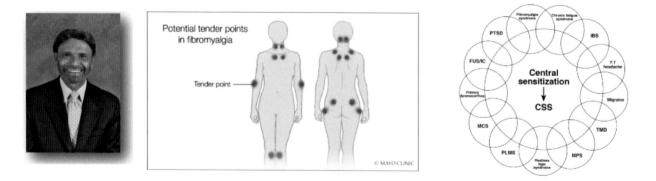

Figure 1: Graphic depicting trigger points associated with fibromyalgia.
Figure 2; Diagram of disorders related to central sensitivity syndrome.

DOB & Place: March 1, 1942, Barishal, Bangladesh

Residence: Peoria, Illinois

Did you know many clinicians initially ignored fibromyalgia and central sensitivity disorders? Before fibromyalgia was more deeply investigated, many rheumatologists considered it a fringe disorder with its exact cause still unknown. Fibromyalgia is one of the most diagnosed chronic pain conditions, affecting ten million Americans and 3–6 percent of the world's population. Dr. Muhammad Yunus made fundamental contributions to the studies of this disorder, beginning with his classic paper published in 1981 that stimulated widespread research interest in this disorder. He is known as the father of the modern view of fibromyalgia. He coined the term central sensitivity syndromes, which refers to a set of disorders, such as irritable bowel syndrome, migraine, and restless legs syndrome, that are related to fibromyalgia. Dr. Yunus is the author of over 100 journal articles with many original contributions and seventeen book chapters and is currently a professor emeritus at the University of Illinois College of Medicine in Peoria. He is an internationally recognized researcher and international speaker in fibromyalgia and related conditions. Dr. Yunus and his collaborators published the first family study with HLA (i.e., tissue) typing of Reiter syndrome (a type of arthritis), the first controlled study of the spectrum of clinical features of fibromyalgia, the first controlled study of juvenile fibromyalgia, the first controlled study of fibromyalgia among the elderly, the first controlled and blind study of muscle biopsy in fibromyalgia, and the first genetic-linkage analysis of multi-case families with fibromyalgia, among others.

Dr. Yunus and his colleagues were also the first to publish a set of data-based criteria for fibromyalgia used nationally and worldwide. They engaged in a heavy scientific debate on the existence of central sensitivity syndromes, a constellation of conditions most physicians now embrace. The majority of those affected by fibromyalgia are women who complained of widespread severe pain, severe fatigue, nonrestorative sleep and sore muscles and joints, among other symptoms. "Doctors back then said, 'They cannot handle life, they are full of stress,'" recalled Dr. Yunus. The FDA now has approved three drugs specifically for the treatment of fibromyalgia: Lyrica (pregabalin), duloxetine (Cymbalta), and milnacipran HCL (Savella). Dr. Yunus's research has made a huge contribution to rheumatology, and he is now well known nationally and internationally in the scientific community.

Frederick Akbar Mohamed

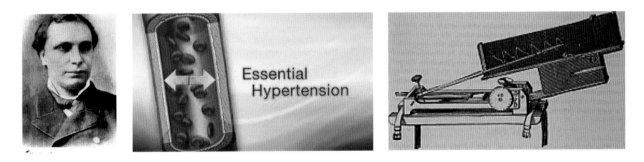

Figure 1; Illustration showing the effects on vessels under high blood pressure.
Figure 2; Figure of Mahomed's modified quantitative sphygmogram.

DOB & Place: April 11, 1849, Brighton, England

Death & Location: November 22, 1884, London, England

Did you know that blood pressure was not recognized as a major measure of heart health until the late nineteenth century? Blood pressure is one of the most fundamental concepts in medicine. It is one of the most common and widely monitored and important vital signs measured in clinical settings and is of critical importance for a physician when assessing a patient's heart health. High blood pressure affects nearly 30 percent of Americans and nearly 26 percent of the world population. The concept of blood pressure was mostly used to assess kidney disorders up until the late nineteenth century. Intriguingly, the first description of blood pressure as a measure/sign of cardiovascular ailments was by a British Muslim physician, Frederick Akbar Mohamed. This concept was not yet known in the 1800s when then medical student Frederick Akbar Mohamed not only discovered the concept of essential hypertension – elevated blood pressure without kidney dysfunction – but also invented one of the earliest practical instruments to measure blood pressure. In his day, it was thought that blood pressure was elevated only due to kidney disease. He was the first to discover that elevated blood pressure is much more prevalent than what was once thought.

Dr. Mohamed, born in Brighton, England, was the son of Saki Dean Mohamed, one of the early Indian immigrants to Britain. His father, a notable entrepreneur, introduced scalp massage (champna), shampoo, and Indian cuisine to the country through his restaurant. Despite facing prejudice and xenophobia as a perceived foreigner, Dr. Frederick Akbar Mohamed made remarkable contributions during his time as a medical student. Notably, he brought attention to elevated blood pressure and raised awareness using a modified tool of his own innovation, the quantitative sphygmogram.

His blood pressure measuring device has since been replaced by the modern blood pressure cuff or sphygmomanometer. Dr. Mohamed classified and described essential hypertension (high blood pressure) in such a critical manner that many contemporaries still hold his older research in high regard. He additionally contributed to advances in blood transfusion and appendectomies for appendicitis. Moreover, he established an organization that would go on to be a guide for the design and methodology of modern clinical trials. Despite the brevity of his career, Mohamed emerged as a trailblazer in his field and an understated contributor to medicine.

Kazi Mobin-Uddin

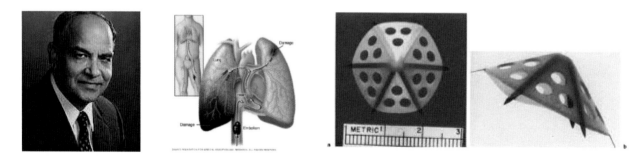

Figure 1; Graphic depicting the damaging effects of pulmonary embolisms.
Figure 2; Pictures of the Uddin Umbrella of Life.

DOB & Place: July 16, 1930, Skindarabad, India

Death & Location: June 10, 1999, Columbus, Ohio

Has anyone heard of an inferior vena cava filter for the treatment of pulmonary embolism? Pulmonary embolisms are a life-threatening condition with 10–30 percent of cases being fatal within the first month of diagnosis. Patients at risk for this condition are those with deep vein thrombosis, another condition in which blood clots form in the lower limbs, which effects an estimated 900,000 Americans per year. A blood clot that forms in the lower extremities and travels to the blood vessels in the lungs, where it block blood flow, is known by the medical term pulmonary embolus (i.e., broken off clot). A pulmonary embolism blocks the lungs from oxygenating (delivering oxygen to the body) and, depending on the severity and treatment, can even lead to death. Pulmonary emboli (plural) rank as the third most common cause of death related to cardiovascular disease, following heart attacks and strokes.

Dr. Kazi Mobin-Uddin, a cardiovascular surgeon, was one of the first to conceive of and develop an implantable inferior vena cava filter that filters blood and blocks the passage of pulmonary emboli. This filter is implanted in patients using a catheter that is inserted in the inferior vena cava (the largest vein in the body that is in the abdomen) and without the need for open surgery. This device was the first FDA-approved commercially available percutaneous IVC filter device (meaning it did not require a large surgical incision).

The inferior vena cava filter is a fundamental device used by physicians for preventing death from pulmonary embolism. Over one million Americans received an IVC filter between 2005 and 2015. Due to the impact of his invention, many in his field consider Dr. Mobin-Uddin the father of modern endovascular surgery. Endovascular surgery revolutionized the fields of surgery, radiology and cardiology by allowing small catheter-based devices/techniques (such a balloon angioplasty and stenting) to replace open cardiac and vascular surgery. Although he is best known for the invention of the IVC filter, Mobin-Uddin also made contributions to the research of myocardial infarctions (heart attacks), coronary revascularization (restoring blood flow), the use of implantable pacemakers, and pulmonary complications of acute pancreatitis. Dr. Mobin-Uddin was also a prolific writer, publishing numerous articles and chapters, and producing well into his retirement up until his death.

Mehmet Oz

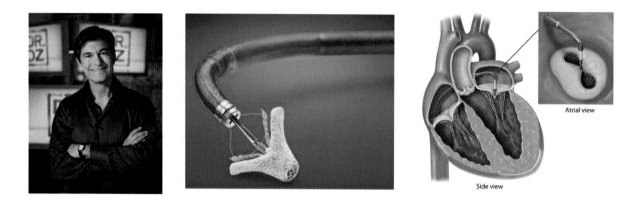

Figure 1: Illustration of the MitralClip.
Figure 2: Illustrated view of the placement of the MitralClip.

DOB & Place: June 11, 1960, Cleveland, Ohio
Residence: Cliffside Park, New Jersey

Who has heard of mitral valve failure? The mitral valve is a heart valve between the left atrium and left ventricle. Failure/regurgitation of this valve is the most common heart valve disorder. Mitral valve insufficiency/disease affects many elderly aged eighty years or older. Mitral valve prolapse affects 2–3 percent of the population, with 176 million worldwide cases and 7.8 million in the United States alone. A lot of people know Dr. Mehmet Oz from his TV show, but he also was the inventor of the percutaneous minimally invasive MitraClip device that many physicians would say was his most fundamental contribution to medicine in addition to the public health awareness he raises through his various widely viewed platforms.

While attending a conference in Italy, Dr. Oz was inspired to create the device from a procedure in the very last portion of the conference. During his flight back to the United States, he formulated a device that would help with mitral valve insufficiency, and he would go on to patent the E-Clip, which later changed to the MitraClip. The MitraClip is a way to use a catheter to treat mitral valve insufficiency with mitral valve prolapse. It allows doctors to treat a condition that is even more common than aortic valve insufficiency or stenosis, which can currently be treated with transcatheter aortic valve replacement (TAVR).

Dr. Oz is also known for patents related to aortic valve replacement and for the Left Ventricular Assist Device (LVADS, a mechanical device that keeps a patient's heart beating while they are waiting for a transplant). Additionally, Dr. Oz is a political activist and was a national senate candidate from Pennsylvania.

Arshad Quadri

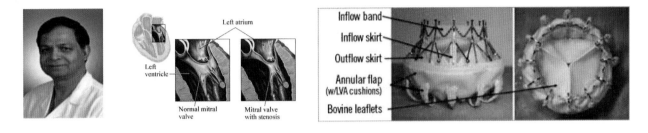

Figure 1; Illustration demonstrating a dysfunctional mitral valve.
Figure 2; Picture of the percutaneous mitral valve replacement prosthesis.

DOB & Place: May 5, 1952, Gaya, India

Residence: West Hartford, Connecticut

Did you know that certain heart valves can be replaced without major surgeries? Dr. Arshad Quadri invented the technology of minimally invasive endovascular mitral and tricuspid valve replacement surgery. Historically, mitral and tricuspid valve surgery is very involved and requires opening the entire chest (i.e., open thoracotomy). Like Dr. Oz's invention, Dr. Quadri's devices are poised to revolutionize the field in light of the previous need for involved surgery.

His first groundbreaking invention was the percutaneous mitral valve, which can be implanted by using a catheter placed into the groin and performed by an interventional cardiologist. This was all done in his garage. His company CardiAQ Valve Technologies was recently acquired by Edwards Lifesciences for $400 million in 2015. Dr. Quadri was able to accomplish this feat despite the fact he did not have the immense resources that universities and other major medical companies have, which are usually necessary to accomplish impactful work (e.g., large laboratories, testing centers, and large sources of funding). This paucity of resources made his achievements that much more astonishing.

His tricuspid valve replacement device is known as the MonarQ Valve which has also been acquired by another medical device company (Peija Medical Inc.) for over $160M. Both his mitral valve and tricuspid valves are undergoing human clinical trials with the first mitral valve implanted in Europe in 2012 and the first tricuspid valve implanted in 2021.

Dr. Quadri continues to innovate with more inventions forthcoming to advance patient cardiovascular care.

Adel Mahmoud

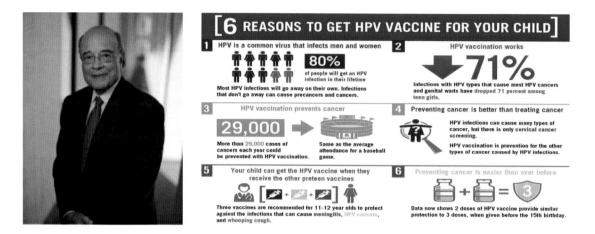

Figure 1: Infographic depicting the benefits of the HPV vaccine.

DOB & Place: August 24, 1941, Cairo, Egypt

Death & Location: June 11, 2018, New York, New York

Does anyone know that a Muslim was responsible for the HPV vaccine? The human papilloma virus (HPV) is a virulent infectious disease that has the potential to cause several types of cancers (e.g., cervical, penile, oral, and anal). This virus is responsible for 12 percent of all cancers and 70 percent of cervical cancers in women. Around fourteen million cases of HPV are diagnosed each year in the United States.

The widely used HPV vaccine was created by Dr. Adel Mahmoud. Dr. Mahmoud was obsessed with infectious diseases and went on to direct Merck Vaccines from 1998 to 2006, where he was responsible for developing many vaccines for viruses such as shingles, rotavirus, and measles/mumps/rubella, in addition to the HPV vaccine. He was also a driving force behind treating Ebola via vaccine before his death. After the Ebola outbreaks in the mid-2010s, Dr. Mahmoud advocated for a global front for vaccine development to help tackle global epidemics. Despite pushback against his attempts to bring various vaccines to market, Dr. Mahmoud prevailed in his struggles and helped save countless lives with his efforts.

Elias Zerhouni

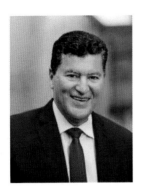
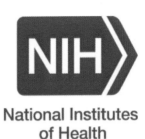

DOB & Place: April 12, 1951, Nedroma, Algeria
Residence: Pasadena, Maryland

Did you know the National Institutes of Health (NIH) was headed by a Muslim physician? The NIH is one of the top biomedical research institutions, ranked only behind Harvard. The NIH had an annual budget of $31.3 billion in 2016. Dr. Zerhouni, who arrived in the United States as an immigrant from Algeria with a limited knowledge of English, and eventually earned a full professorship at Johns Hopkins University, one of the most prestigious medical schools in the world.

Specializing in magnetic resonance imaging (MRI) and computed tomography (CT), he made seminal contributions in his field, becoming an internationally recognized leader/expert in radiological imaging. He pioneered many uses of MRI technology, thus revolutionizing the ways in which it could be applied to diagnosing cardiovascular diseases and cancer. He introduced a molecular-tagging system that allowed for a noninvasive method of tracking three-dimensional motions of the heart. Additionally, he was renowned for helping create a CT imaging system to identify cancerous masses, specifically aiding with the early diagnosis of breast cancers. Dr. Zerhouni's academic career was spent at Johns Hopkins Hospital, where he was professor of radiology and biomedical engineering and senior advisor for Johns Hopkins Medicine.

In addition to serving as a consultant to the White House and to President Ronald Reagan in 1985, he assisted in establishing the Institute for Cell Engineering at Johns Hopkins. He performed his duties as the chair of the Russell H. Morgan Department of Radiology and Radiological Sciences, vice dean of research, and the executive vice dean of the School of Medicine from 1996 to 2002 before his appointment as director of the NIH by President George W. Bush between 2002 and 2008. Dr. Zerhouni was heralded as an excellent administrator at both Johns Hopkins and the NIH, establishing numerous programs that helped increase the status of medical research and raise public health awareness. Overseeing the NIH Roadmap for Medical Research, he helped accelerate the course of critical studies and provide valuable needed funds. He was also a proponent of studying public health disparities, making it a priority to uncover disease burden discrepancies through collaborations with other research facilities.

In November 2009, President Barack Obama appointed Dr. Zerhouni as one of the first presidential US science envoys. Dr. Zerhouni also served as senior fellow to the Bill and Melinda Gates Foundation from 2009 to 2010 and senior advisor to the CEO of the French pharmaceutical company Sanofi (stepping down as head of global research and development in 2018). Dr. Zerhouni has founded or cofounded five startup companies, authored more than 200 publications, and received several patents. He has taken positions on several boards, including most recently, the boards of the Lasker Foundation, Research!America, and the NIH Foundation. He was also chosen as a member of the US National Academy of Medicine and the US National Academy of Engineering. He was awarded the prestigious Legion of Honor medal from the French National Order in 2008 and was elected in 2010 as a member of the French Academy of Medicine, as well as being appointed chair of innovation at the College de France in 2011. Dr. Zerhouni was a remarkable administrator and contributor to medical sciences, making tremendous advantages in his field and medical research in general. This medical thought leader is an intrepid and collaborative leader with a multidisciplinary approach and transformative thinking.

Amir Motarjeme

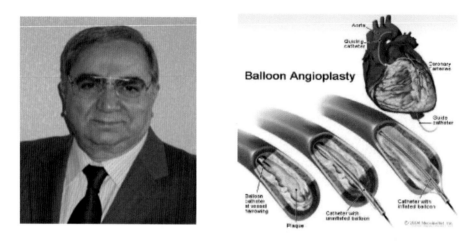

Figure I; Graphic showing how a transluminal balloon angioplasty can open an occluded blood vessel.

DOB & Place: March 17, 1937, Iran

Residence: Downers Grove, Illinois

Percutaneous transluminal angioplasty, or balloon angioplasty, is one of the most fundamental life-saving contributions to medicine. Every year, more than one million Americans undergo a balloon angioplasty. It is used in all sorts of vascular and nonvascular conditions throughout the body and wherever luminal narrowing occurs. The technique basically involves inflating a balloon under high pressure to dilate a tubular structure or opening.

It is integral to stenting, the treatment of heart attacks and preventing amputations, as well as for dialysis patients. This procedure is one of the most commonly used and fundamental endovascular techniques to open blocked blood vessels (i.e., arteries and veins). Dr. Motarjeme was a major developer of percutaneous transluminal angioplasty. Recently in an article in the Journal of Vascular and Interventional Radiology about the history of interventional radiology titled "The Early Years.", Dr. Amir Motarjeme was listed as one of the seven pioneers of percutaneous transluminal angioplasty.

For vascular interventionists, he was the major thought leader in the field throughout his career. He was also one of the first to host an endovascular conference for treatment of peripheral (outside of the heart) arterial disease. His technical skill set was not only innovative but legendary. On a related note, Dr. Motarjeme also pioneered the use of clot-dissolving drugs (i.e., thrombolytics) in lower extremity interventions throughout the body.

Alam Nisar Syed

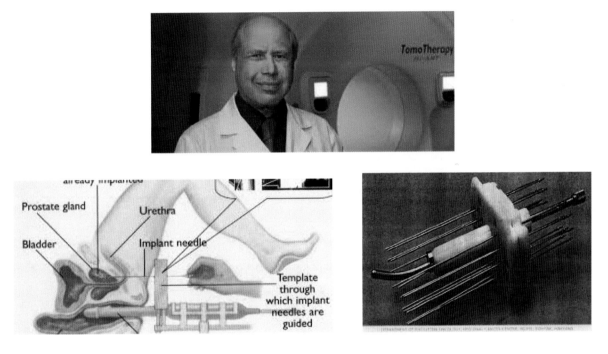

Figure 1: Illustration demonstrating an interstitial brachytherapy treatment through a Seed Implant.
Figure 2: Picture of a seed implant for brachytherapy.

DOB & Place: August 1, 1940, Karimnagar, India
Residence: Long Beach, California

Cancer is one of the most feared diagnoses anyone could have. Has anyone heard of brachytherapy treatment for prostate and cervical cancers? Every year, nearly two million people in the United States and more than eighteen million people worldwide are diagnosed with cancer, the most common being lung, breast, skin, prostate, cervical, and rectal cancers. Dr. Alam Nisar Syed single-handedly created the entire field of interstitial brachytherapy, with his innovative inventions and techniques.

His seed implants are routinely used throughout the world as an effective minimally invasive treatment for prostate, cervical, and related cancers (e.g., head/neck, skin, breast, gallbladder, uterine, vaginal, lung, rectal, and eye). These implants emit localized, high-dose (cancer-killing) radiation directly to the tumor without the complications/invasive nature of radical surgery and the adverse effects of external beam radiation or systemic chemotherapy. His cost-effective approach has revolutionized the treatment of these common types of cancers. Dr. Syed's influence resonates across the field of brachytherapy, as he has trained over 2,000 physicians with his life-saving procedures. Additionally, he founded the American Society for Brachytherapy and established the Journal of Brachytherapy, showcasing his steadfast dedication to sustaining and advancing his field of medicine.

Muhammad Mansoor Mohiuddin

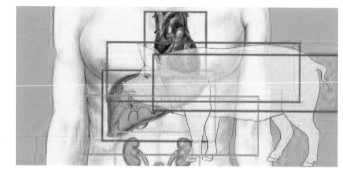

DOB & Place: August 9, 1964, Hyderabad, India
Residence: Maryland

In 2022, a groundbreaking headline announced the first successful transplantation of a genetically engineered pig heart into a terminally ill human. The first patient survived only sixty days due to his underlying frail state and immunosuppression, However, this medical breakthrough, known as xenotransplantations (the transplantation of animal organs into a human), is a potential solution to the organ transplant shortage affecting more than one hundred thousand Americans on waiting lists. Over six thousand of these patients die every year due to the lack of available donor organs.

The xenotransplantation was possible only through the pioneering efforts of Dr. Mohiuddin who in 1992 confounded the University of Maryland program that worked on this project. In 2014, he first demonstrated that genetically altered pig hearts can survive as long as three years when implanted in the abdomen of a baboon. His team therefore holds the record of longest xenograft survival in a large animal model. Additionally, the immunosuppressive regimen developed under his leadership is now used widely throughout the xenotransplantation field. Dr. Mohiuddin had previously served as Chief of Transplantation at the NIH's Cardiothoracic Surgery Research Program as well as a Senior Scientist at the National Heart Lung and Blood Institute of the NIH.

Teepu Siddique

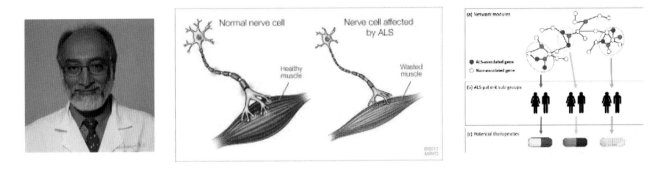

**Figure 1: Illustration demonstrating the effects of ALS on individual muscle fibers.
Figure 2: Graphic showing molecular/genetic divisions of
patient's with muscular degenerative diseases.**

DOB & Place: December 2, 1947, Lahore, Pakistan

Residence: Chicago, Illinois

Amyotrophic lateral sclerosis (ALS) is one of the most debilitating and researched diseases of the modern era. This neurological condition has stricken many major public figures, including the brilliant physicist Stephen Hawking and the legendary baseball player Lou Gehrig. ALS has been in the public eye for many decades. Awareness of ALS has been popularized with viral campaigns such as the ALS Ice Bucket Challenge, but the exact cause and effective treatment of this devastating disease still remains a mystery.

However, one of the most seminal discoveries required for identifying effective future treatments of ALS was the identification of the genetic factors that cause and promote the disease. This discovery was made by Dr. Teepu Siddique who uncovered and identified the major genetic components behind ALS. Dr. Siddique has actually been heralded by his esteemed peers as a future Nobel Prize winner. Through his research he was able to describe the three major genes that are likely responsible for ALS and at the same time identified corresponding drugs that could effectively treat it.

Dr. Siddique has also made critical advances in the general study of ALS, establishing a reliable animal model for future ALS researchers. He has also made fundamental contributions to the genetic causes of Duchenne muscular dystrophy (a disease involving progressive weakening of the muscles), spastic paraplegia (a disease-causing paralysis with spasms), and inherited neuropathy (a disease of the nerves). Dr. Siddique's brilliant discoveries have cemented him as part of the foundation for the research and treatment of muscular degenerative diseases.

Huda Zoghbi

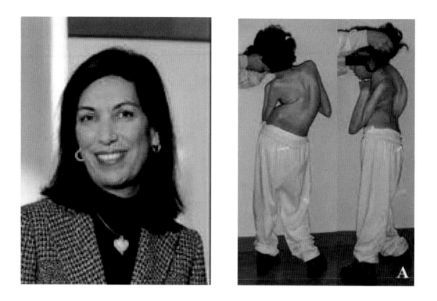

Figure I: 15-year-old female with Rett Syndrome and severe scoliosis

DOB & Place: June 20th, 1954, Beirut, Lebanon

Residence: Houston, Texas

Neurological diseases are devastating conditions especially in children. It would be interesting to know that a Muslim physician has made great strides in decoding the genetic origins of these diseases. Dr. Huda Zoghbi is a prolific researcher in genetics and neuroscience, making foundational discoveries in the genetic origins of Rett syndrome (a developmental disorder, mostly affecting young girls that can lead to regression and disability), spinocerebellar ataxia (SCA, a disorder that involves progressive loss of balance and coordination, as well as swallowing difficulties), and a childhood brain cancer called medulloblastoma. Her discoveries have given researchers and physicians potential new pathways to treat patients afflicted with these disorders.

Like quite of few of the physicians in this chapter she managed to escape her war-torn nation in this case during the Lebanese civil war while a medical student at the prestigious American University of Beirut. Dr. Zoghbi pursued her pediatric residency at Baylor College of Medicine in Houston, Texas, and chose to remain there. She rose to the position of Chief Pediatrics Resident and later specialized in Pediatric Neurology. In 1985, the year she attained U.S. citizenship and was expecting her first child, Dr. Zoghbi faced the heart-wrenching task of informing parents about their children's severe genetic disorders. She published a paper describing Rett's syndrome and developed expertise in diagnosing this disease, but also realized that this disease likely had a genetic basis. Motivated to make a difference, yet with no prior training in molecular biology, she delved into molecular genetics research, aiming to understand and potentially eliminate some of these neurological diseases.

She made her groundbreaking discovery of the SCA causing gene (ATAXIN1) in 1993 while pursuing her research into the causes of Rett syndrome. Only six years later, Dr. Zoghbi was able to identify another gene (MECP2) as the cause of Rett syndrome, more importantly her findings established a straightforward genetic test to diagnose Rett syndrome early and more accurately.

Her research showed the brain's sensitivity to MeCP2 protein levels, produced by the MECP2 gene. Insufficient MeCP2 leads to Rett syndrome, while excess results in neurological deficits and the MECP2 duplication syndrome. MECP2 mutations can also cause conditions from autism to juvenile schizophrenia. Her insights proved that some autism and intellectual disabilities can be genetic without being inherited.

Dr. Zoghbi's research was so profound that it contributed to the start of a new field of study: the role of epigenetics (how control of gene expression affects genetic traits, rather than just the genetic code itself) in neuropsychiatric disorders. In 2010, Dr. Zoghbi established the Neurological Research Institute at Texas Children's Hospital. Over the years, her exemplary work in genetics and neuroscience has earned her numerous accolades, including the Kavli prize from Norway in 2022 and the Breakthrough Award presented by Mark Zuckerberg and Sergey Brin in 2017.

Jihad Mustapha and Fadi Saab

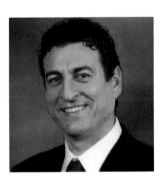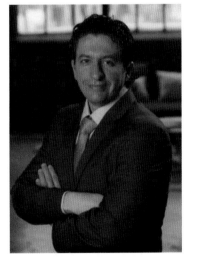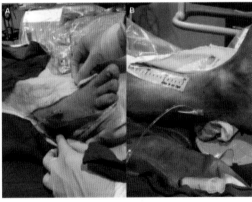

Caption: Image depicting direct access/puncture of the pedal arteries for lower extremity intervention.

DOB & Place: June 10, 1967, Tyre, Lebanon
Residence: Grand Rapids, Michigan

DOB & Place: November 26, 1975, Kuwait City, Kuwait
Residence: Grand Rapids, Michigan

Did you know that the lack of blood flow to a limb could lead to an amputation? Amputations are often due to inadequate blood supply to the lower extremities in a condition called critical limb ischemia (CLI). This is typically due to peripheral arterial disease which is explained in detail in the previous section (see Amman Bolia). It has been reported that up to twenty-nine percent of patients with CLI will either have an amputation or die within the first year of their diagnosis. For patients with CLI-related amputations the five year mortality rate is up to fifty-six percent, a rate higher than many common forms of cancer. The treatment is to restore the blood flow, which reduces the rate of death by half when compared to amputation. Dr. Jihad Mustapha developed a new way to restore blood flow (without surgery) to prevent amputations.

Dr. Mustapha's journey to prominence began when he fled war-torn western Lebanon at the age of fifteen and arrived in New York City, unfamiliar with the English language. From selling umbrellas on the street to working as a busboy and undertaking janitorial duties, his perseverance led him to attend medical school in the Caribbean. Today, he is internationally recognized as a pioneering authority on CLI treatment to prevent amputations, earning him the moniker "the leg saver."

He introduced the transpedal arterial minimally invasive procedure, a technique that addresses arterial blockages in the legs when conventional treatments fail. This method involves directly puncturing arteries in the foot to reopen blockages and restore circulation. Notably, Dr. Mustapha organizes one of the largest gatherings focused on amputation prevention—the Amputation Prevention Symposium (AMP). The 2018 conference boasted over 1,000 physicians in attendance. A prolific speaker, Dr. Mustapha is consistently associated with cutting-edge studies and groundbreaking innovations in the field of peripheral arterial disease treatments.

It's essential to acknowledge the significant contributions of Dr. Fadi Saab, a longtime collaborator of Dr. Jihad Mustapha and co-director of the AMP conference. Dr. Saab is a respected expert and thought leader in his own right regarding CLI. Witnessing the limited attention given to CLI patients at other institutions, these physicians established an independent CLI center named Advanced Cardiac and Vascular Amputation Prevention Centers (ACV). This dedicated center focuses on treating at-risk CLI patients and quickly demonstrated its necessity by reaching operational capacity within nine months. "We believe the center that we've created is providing a much-needed service for patients with this deadly disease," says Dr. Saab. "We feel that this model [including hardware and the team] can be replicated in other locations around the country." Dr. Saab is also a prolific presenter/panelist at many international conferences regarding peripheral vascular disease and CLI. He is also a frequent presenter and panelist at international conferences addressing peripheral vascular disease and CLI.

Mark S. Humayun

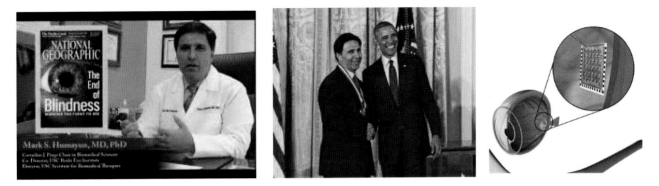

DOB & Place: August 3rd 1962, Pakistan

Residence: San Diego, CA

Over one million people in the United States suffer from blindness. During the 1970s, a television series called "The Six Million Dollar Man" showcased an astronaut possessing superhuman abilities after receiving bionic legs, a right arm, and a right eye as part of his reconstruction. Interestingly, in present times, a real-life bionic eye has been developed by a Muslim inventor.

Dr. Mark Humayun invented the world's first artificial retina (the part of the rear of the eye that is the most complex and is like a screen that transmits images to the brain) as part of a thirty-year effort. His Argus II retinal implant provides vision to someone with complete blindness. It was approved by the FDA in 2013. Dr. Humayun was inspired to pursue ophthalmology after his grandmother lost her sight to diabetes. As both an ophthalmologist and a biomedical engineer at the University of Southern California, he assembled a world class interdisciplinary team of biomedical engineers, computer scientists, chemists, biologists, and business experts to create the first artificial retina. The device works by taking an image from a tiny video camera and transmitting it wirelessly as electrical signals to tiny electrodes implanted on the surface of the patient's retina. The light stimulation pattern is then recognized as vision in the patient's brain. It allows patients to read and walk outside with further improvements to come.

He has more than 125 granted patents and has been elected as a fellow in the Academy of Inventors. He was also elected to the prestigious National Academy of Medicine (NAM) and National Academy of Engineering (NAE) for his pioneering work to restore sight. He has received several awards for this, including the 2005 Innovator of the Year Award. He was also featured as one of the top ten inventors by Time magazine in 2013. In 2016 he received the National Medal of Technology and Innovation from President Barack Obama for his work in developing the Argus II. The Argus award distinguishes those who have made lasting contributions to America's competitiveness and quality of life and helped strengthen the nation's technological workforce He also received the 2018 Institute of Electrical and Electronics Engineers (IEEE) Biomedical Engineering Award. Additionally, he was awarded the 2020 IEEE Medal for Innovations in Healthcare Technology.

Abdul Mateen Ahmed

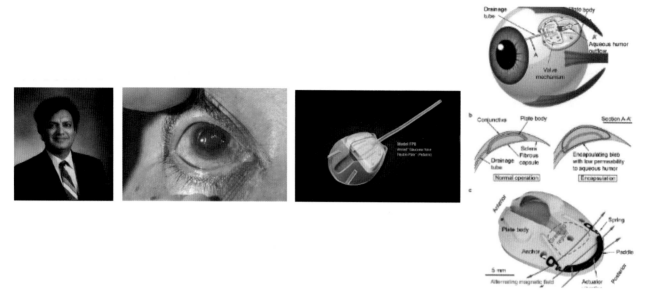

Figure 1: Picture of a patient with glaucoma.
Figure 2-4: Illustration of the Ahmed Glaucoma Valve.

DOB & Place: March 27, 1944, Wani, India
Residence: Rancho Cucamonga, California

Do you know what is the most common cause of blindness? Glaucoma is the world's leading cause of permanent blindness. It is due to elevated pressure from excessive fluid inside the eyeball within the anterior chamber of the eye, which lies directly behind the cornea. The pressure caused by this fluid buildup is transmitted all the way through the rest of the eye (posterior and vitreous chambers) and back to the optic nerve, leading to damage and eventual blindness. Dr. Ahmed invented what is called the Ahmed Glaucoma Valve, which treats glaucoma by draining the excessive fluid. In fact, this is now the standard treatment for glaucoma.

He was inspired to create this device when other medications failed during a stint in Nigeria. Interestingly, the previously mentioned ailment river blindness was pervasive in Nigeria increasing the number of cases of glaucoma. His device has been so successful that it has actually captured around seventy percent of the world market for glaucoma valves.

Madjid Samii

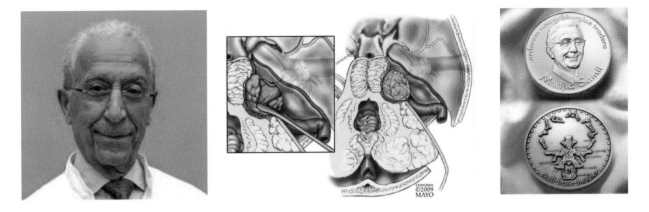

Figure: Illustration of a cerebellopontine angle vestibular schwannoma.

DOB & Place: June 19th, 1937 Tehran, Iran
Residence: Hannover, Germany

Did you know there was a physician who is considered instrumental to the development of modern neurosurgery? Neurosurgery giant Dr. Majid Samii is widely regarded as a foremost expert in the field, founding many societies and conferences for the dissemination of the newest developments in the field, including serving as the president of the International Society for Neurosurgery. He made key advancements in operating microscopic tools for neurosurgery. Dr. Samii's work has been so impactful that in 2011 the World Federation of Neurosurgical Societies coined a medal in his name to be given to a distinguished neurosurgeon every two years. One of his major achievements was pioneering the safe operative removal of a brain tumor called a vestibular schwannoma or acoustic neuroma from a particular difficult area of the skull to remove (called the cerebellopontine angle).

It has been said that his research on acoustic neuroma's (a common type of benign brain tumor, causing deafness and loss of balance) "will remain fundamental literature on the issue for future generations. His contribution to the knowledge of this disease is considered the gold standard to which every modern neurosurgeon has to aspire. However, there is no specific aspect of neurosurgery that has not received his innovative signature". One of the most revered neurosurgeons in history honored Dr. Samii stating "[his] surgical dexterity, his falcon-like mental eye, and his strong will and stamina established him as a world-renowned neurosurgeon". Another one of his esteemed neurosurgical peer described him as "one of the greatest neurosurgeon to walk the earth".

A prolific educator Dr. Samii established the first course on skull-based surgeries in the early 1970's. His passion for educating future neurosurgeons is continuously honored by numerous national and international awards throughout the world. Dr. Samii was the editor of many prestigious journals, and has received many honorary doctorates and professorships.

Moncef Saloui

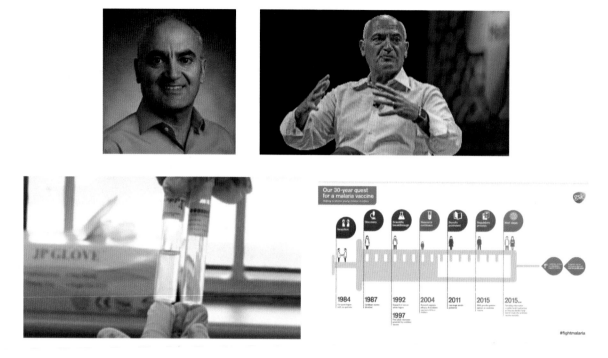

DOB & Place: July 22, 1959, Agadir, Morocco
Residence: Greater Philadelphia, PA

A major focus during the global COVID-19 pandemic was the search for a vaccine. Do you know who was the leader of the US effort to invent the vaccine? Dr. Moncef Saloui, a molecular biologist and immunologist, as well as Muslim immigrant from Morocco, was the first choice to lead the deployment of Operation Warp Speed; the federal initiative to accelerate the development of COVID-19 vaccines. Of note, the second choice was the formerly recognized Dr. Elias Zerhouni.

Dr. Saloui is an established researcher and former professor at the University of Mons (Belgium). He first came to the United States when he took postgraduate courses at Harvard and Tufts School of Medicine. Dr. Saloui has also been responsible for efforts that have produced other notable vaccines, including Cervarix to prevent cervical cancer, Rotarix prevention of rotavirus-induced gastroenteritis (causing severe diarrhea and vomiting in infants and children), the Ebola virus, Synflorix to prevent pneumococcal diseases (e.g., pneumonia and meningitis), and Mosquitrix the first ever malaria vaccine. He founded the Saloui Center for Vaccines Research in Rockville, Maryland, in 2016 and was touted by Alex Azar, the secretary of Health and Human Services, as "arguably the world's most experienced and successful vaccine developer."

Ozlem Tureci and Ugur Sahin

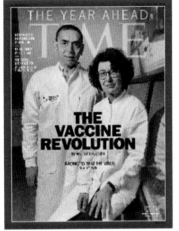
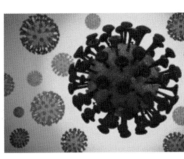
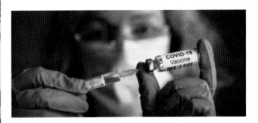

DOB & Place: March 7th 1967, Lastrup, Germany

DOB & Place: September 29,1965 Iskenderun, Turkey

Do you know who developed the world first mRNA COVID vaccine? Ozlem Tureci and Ugur Sahin were the power couple behind the development of the world's first messenger RNA based COVID-19 vaccine going from laboratory and clinical testing to conditional approval within a record 11 months. Ozlem Tureci an immunologist is the chief medical officer of BioNTech which she cofounded with her husband Ugur Sahin, oncologist and CEO of BioNTech. Both have had a distinguished career in teaching and research before founding two pharmaceutical companies. The first one they sold (Ganymed Pharmaceuticals in 2016 for $1.4B) and the second one after its 2019 IPO was worth over $21 B in November 2020. They are currently developing immune therapy based cancer vaccines with the start of human testing in Britain.

It is only fitting that Muslims are some of the world's leaders in developing vaccines, as the world has come full circle in that Muslims in the Islamic Golden Age pioneered the concept of acquired immunity (Al Rhazes in the 8th century), and later on routinely practiced an effective precursor to vaccination for smallpox. In fact, the technique of inoculation was introduced by European physicians and scientists, based on their observations of this routine practice in the Ottoman Empire.

HONORABLE MENTIONS

Syed Modasser Ali

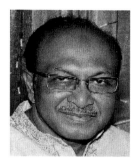

Syed Modasser Ali is on the list of the 20 most innovative surgeons of the world. He is an ophthalmologist and a preeminent administrator in the Bangladeshi government. He was a physician of many firsts: writing a textbook on public eye health in 1985 entitled Community Ophthalmology (recognized as the first textbook on the subject by the British Journal of Ophthalmology), opening the first eye hospital in Bangladesh and helped establish the first peer-reviewed ophthalmology journal in Bangladesh.

Dr. Ali's ingenuity and passion for public health has led him to be a pioneer in community eye health and general health, globally. He was chosen to be an Executive Board Member of the World Health Organization (WHO). Dr. Ali also became the director-general for the department of public health of Bangladesh. Through his many public health endeavors and surgical innovations, Dr. Ali is regarded as a revolutionary force for advancing medical sciences and healthcare.

Mahmood Hai

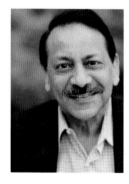

Mahmood Hai is a urologist who is internationally renowned for his pioneering work on Green light laser devices. Dr. Hai was the leader of a clinical trial collaboration with the Mayo Clinic under the FDA, which was the first to implement Green light laser technology to treat prostate blockages. Green light laser technology can restore natural urine flow within twenty-four hours and has revolutionized prostate surgery. He has trained thousands of urologists around the world and the procedure has been performed in over one million patients. Contributing to hundreds of publications, he is widely acknowledged as he is often called upon to perform surgeries on various diplomats, celebrities, and world leaders. Based in Michigan, Dr. Hai helped establish the Michigan Education Council in 1991 and has been recognized for his many philanthropic and interfaith outreach programs.

Resad Pazic

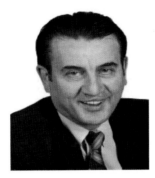

One of the world's foremost specialists in laparoscopic gynecological surgery and the president of the corresponding society is Muslim physician Dr. Resad Pazic. Working out of Louisville, Kentucky, he fled as a refugee from his war-torn home country, Bosnia. Of note, many of the physicians featured in this compilation are refugees.

Jafar Golzarian

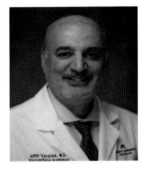

One of the world's experts on embolization, a widely used endovascular technique to intentionally occlude a vessel for many clinical applications, is also Muslim: Dr. Jafar Golzarian. He is a professor of radiology and the director of the Interventional Radiology & Vascular Imaging Department at the University of Minnesota Medical School. He co-founded and is president of the largest meeting for embolization—Global Embolization Symposium & Technologies (GEST)—and the inventor of beads for treatment using embolization procedures. His fundamental research has led to the development of many novel materials and more than 12 patents for many clinical applications. Dr. Golzarian has pioneered the development of many minimally-invasive interventions which include treatments for peripheral arterial disease, treatment for endoleaks (a leakage of blood outside of the stent graft) following an endovascular abdominal aortic aneurysm repair, as well as embolization treatments for uterine fibroids, hepatocellular carcinoma, and benign prostatic hyperplasia (BPH). In addition to authoring over 450 peer-reviewed publications, he has written over 120 peer-reviewed publications, a textbook on Embolotherapy, and more than 14 book chapters.

Husain Sattar

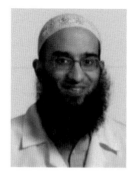

Dr. Sattar, a surgical pathologist, established the Pathoma Course for pathologic learning, one of the most popular online courses for medical students. This course includes a widely successful and effective series of books and videos, which has provided medical students with invaluable information. "He can take the pathophysiology of any organ system and present the information in a way that makes the entire mechanism click in your head. He has this amazing way of explaining concepts … He simplifies things to the most basic elements," stated Lucy Rubin, a fourth-year medical student at Tufts University School of Medicine.

Ghaus Malik

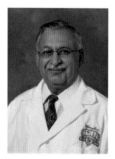

Dr. Ghaus Malik is one of the world's leading authorities in cerebrovascular neurosurgery, especially aneurysms (focal ballooning outpouching of blood vessels that can rupture and cause major death or disability) and arteriovascular malformations (abnormal connections between arteries and veins in the brain or spinal cord that can also rupture) as well as trigeminal neuralgia (pain arising from the nerve supplying the face, jaw, and eyes). His work recently has focused on predicting potential rupture risk of intracranial aneurysm using artificial intelligence and deep learning. He is also considered a master in AVM surgery. His unique and pioneering endeavors on AVMs, involving one of the largest series in the world over the past thirty years, has left an indelible mark on the neurosurgical treatment of this fearful condition. He has published over 113 peer-reviewed articles in his field and has trained over eighty neurosurgeons. He was recognized with the Walter C. Dandy Medal in 2015, the highest honor the Walter E. Dandy Neurosurgical Society bestows upon a neurosurgeon.

Malik Kahook

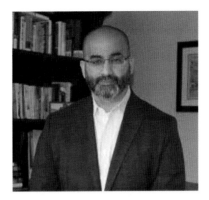

Dr. Kahook is recognized by many in his field for his ingenuity in developing unique devices for the treatment of glaucoma and other ophthalmologic conditions. Inventor of the Kahook blade and Harmoni Intraocular Lens, he holds over sixty patents and is a prolific researcher/author at the University of Colorado School of Medicine.

Nadia Bukhari

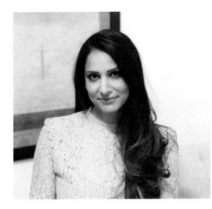

Nadia Bukhari, a respected figure at University College London (UCL), is known as UCL's pharmacy ambassador, advocating for pharmacists' role in healthcare. She's achieved milestones like becoming the youngest female Asian Fellow of the Royal Pharmaceutical Society and the first Muslim woman on England's National Pharmacy Board. A strong supporter of women's rights, she's also active with the Pakistan Alliance for Girls Education (PAGE). Bukhari promotes gender equity among pharmacists nationally and globally, notably with the International Pharmaceutical Federation. Her involvement spans leadership research, mentoring, and chairing conferences. She's also affiliated with Higher Education Academy and Hamdard University, Islamabad.

Afshin Gangi

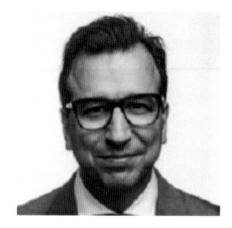

An interventional radiologist in France, Dr. Afshin Gangi is a well-respected authority on cryoablation, or the use of liquid nitrogen–cooled ice rods to freeze/kill tumors, as well as interventional spinal treatments. Dr. Gangi is a prolific speaker, presenter, and author, displaying his passion to spread information on treatments he finds critical for patient health. He has also received the prestigious French award Victoire de la Médecine twice, in 2009 and 2010.

Ahmed Okasha

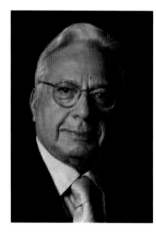

Director of the WHO's Collaborating Center for Training and Research in Mental Health and a professor of psychiatry, Dr. Ahmed Okasha is a foundational figure in mental health and the first Arab Muslim to head the World Psychiatric Organization, as well as a respected author of seminal textbooks for psychiatric training. Dr. Okasha is a preeminent force in advocacy for mental public health and advancing the field of psychiatry.

Muhammad Asim Khan

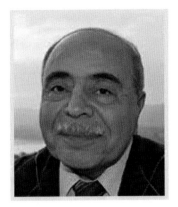

Dr. Muhammad Asim Khan is an internationally renowned expert and lecturer on ankylosing spondylitis, an inflammatory arthritis that can result in joint fusion or ankylosis. He has a personal connection to the disease and is diagnosed with it. Authoring many scientific papers on ankylosing spondylitis and other rheumatology-related articles, Dr. Khan has made significant contributions to public awareness with his book Ankylosing Spondylitis: The Facts.

Azra Raza

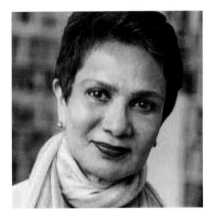

Dr. Azra Raza, a hematology oncologist, has done seminal work in the treatment and research of myelodysplastic syndrome. This disease involves a constellation of symptoms such as anemia, fatigue, and discoloration, and is caused by the dysfunction of blood clot formation. She is also an expert on myeloid leukemia. She also established the MDS tissue bank to study myelodysplastic syndrome. This is a tissue repository holding more than 60,000 samples of myelodysplastic syndrome and myeloid leukemia and is considered a national treasure. She was part of Obama's "cancer moonshot" program, an initiative aimed to cure cancer.

Mahmoud Ghannoum

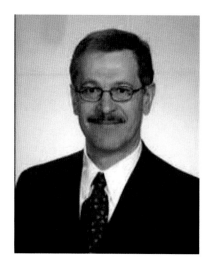

Dr. Mahmoud Ghannoum is widely recognized as the world's leading expert on the microbiome, or the body's collection of gut bacteria, virtually initiating the field of studies on the mycobiome, or the body's collection of gut fungi. Dr. Ghannoum immigrated to the United States in hopes of finding a position, and he would have left despondent had it not been for the kindness of a travel agent who rearranged his travels and lent him money as well. After realizing that current microbiome-nutritional supplements targeted only bacteria, he and his son opened BIOHM, the first company that addresses the gut's total microbiome of both bacteria and fungus.

Mostafa El-Sayed

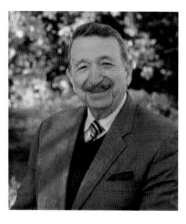

Dr. El-Sayed is an internationally recognized chemist and researcher on the use of nanoparticles to combat cancer. After his wife was diagnosed with breast cancer, he turned his efforts to treat certain cancers with nano-golden rods supplemented with phototherapy. He and his research team made a stunning breakthrough after discovering that certain-sized rods convert light to heat, allowing a new method to possibly kill cancerous tumors.

Mohammed Saiful Huq

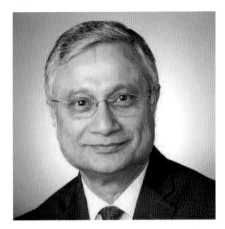

Saiful Haq is a world leader in medical physics. He was elected president of the American Association of Physicists in Medicine in 2020. He has received numerous awards and recognitions for his work, including the Farrington Daniels Award from the AAPM in 1992, which is the highest recognition offered by the journal Medical Physics, for his work in radiation dosimetry showing how measuring the dose with a device called a water calorimeter provides results comparable to an ionization chamber.

He has over 183 publications, close to 7,000 citations, and an h-index of 36 (84 percent of Nobel Prize winners in physics have had an h-index of at least 30). He was the founding member of the editorial board of the Journal of Biomedical Physics and Engineering (2015–2016) and has coauthored two major textbooks in his field, Radiation Oncology Therapy and Stereotactic Radiosurgery and Stereotactic Body Radiation Therapy. He serves as chair of the board of the AAPM and is the director of the Medical Physics Division University of Pittsburgh Cancer Institute, UPMC Cancer Center, Department of Radiation Oncology.

Hamid Ikram

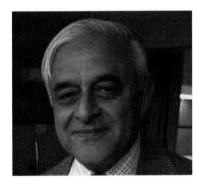

A cardiologist based in New Zealand, Dr. Hamid Ikram has published seminal works that further the understanding of hormonal control over heart functions. Dr. Ikram was a foundational force in establishing critically needed heart services to the residents of Christchurch, New Zealand, as well as Maori natives.

Masood Akhtar

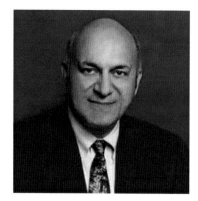

Dr. Akhtar is ranked among the world's preeminent electrophysiologists and has trained hundreds of physicians at the electrophysiology fellowship program he created at the University of Wisconsin in Milwaukee. Dr. Akhtar was a prolific publisher of research on the role and treatment of the sinoatrial node and atrioventricular node on heart rhythms. These nodes are originators and conductors of electrical signals in the heart. He has been listed in "The Best Doctors in America" for several decades. The American Heart Association's Wisconsin affiliate named him cardiovascular researcher of the year in 1984. Harvard Medical school honored him with a memorial lecture in 2019.

Mehdi Shishehbor

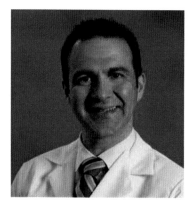

Dr. Mehdi Shishehbor is a key opinion leader in the field of cardiovascular epidemiology and intervention. He is a respected researcher in cardiovascular medicine and interventional cardiology and has won a number of awards at international and national events. He is a cofounder of the international conference Cardiovascular Innovations, one of the largest meetings in interventional cardiology with over 1,500 attendees. He recently in 2023 was the lead author of a landmark article in the prestigious top medical journal New England Journal of Medicine for breakthrough TADAV (transcatheter arterialization of deep veins) procedure where deep veins in the leg and foot are converted into arteries to provide blood flow to prevent amputations in patients who have no surgical or endovascular alternatives.

Alexander Norbash

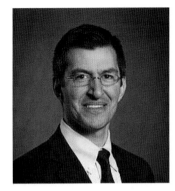

An interventional neuroradiologist, Dr. Norbash helped pioneer the use of stenting for the carotid arteries. Dr. Norbash is a highly regarded clinician and device developer, innovating ultrathin stents for the endovascular treatment of aneurysms, laser-assisted stroke thrombolysis, resorbable polymer stents, injectable polymer and hydrogel vascular embolic occlusive compounds, and operator controllable remote-motion microcatheters.

Khalid Shah

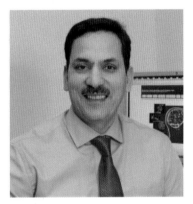

Dr. Shah is the vice chair of research at Brigham Women's Hospital and the director of the Center for Stem Cell Therapeutics and Imaging at Harvard Medical School. He researches new stem-cell therapies to target metastatic brain tumors and is a professor at Harvard Medical School, as well as principal faculty at the Harvard Stem Cell Institute. He directs the joint Center of Excellence in Biomedicine with King Abdulaziz City for Science and Technology, Saudi Arabia. Dr. Shah and his team have advanced the field of stem-cell therapy by creating models to better understand the fundamentals of cancer biology and stem-cell therapeutics.

Recently, Dr. Shah's laboratory has reverse-engineered cancer cells using CRISPR/Cas9 technology and utilized them as therapeutics to treat cancer. This work has garnered attention from mainstream media outlets such as CNN, BBC, NPR, Scientific American and the New York Times. A productive author and sought-after presenter, advisor, international grant reviewer, and mentor, Dr. Shah has published numerous peer-reviewed articles in high-impact journals. He has also written two books and presented at over 300 seminars worldwide. He has founded two biotech companies to treat cancer with therapeutic cellular technology. Currently he holds more than ten patents and has received numerous awards recognizing his innovative and impactful work.

Rozina Ali

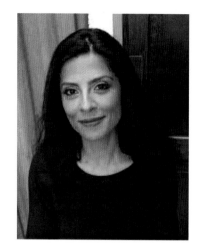

Dr. Rozina Ali is a world-renowned plastic surgeon and public health advocate based in the United Kingdom. She has been leading the advancement of reconstructive surgery in using fat transfer, perforator flaps and microsurgical techniques. Specializing in breast surgery, facial surgery, liposuction and nonsurgical aesthetics, Dr. Ali is a prolific public speaker and author. Appearing in two separate mainstream television programs in the UK (the BBC's documentary 'The Truth about Looking Younger' and Channel 4's series 'How not to get old'), she has raised tremendous amounts of awareness in the fields of breast augmentation, microvascular surgery and reconstructive surgery generally.

Ali Guermazi

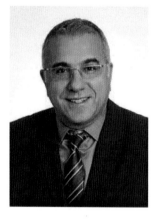

Dr. Ali Guermazi is a highly regarded radiologist and innovator in the diagnosis and disease progression of osteoarthritis through MRI. Having published over 300 peer-reviewed works. Dr. Guermazi has been involved in developing several original and widely accepted radiological methods to assess osteoarthritis disease risk and progression, including the WORMS (whole organ magnetic resonance imaging score), BLOKS (Boston Leeds osteoarthritis knee score), and MOAKS (MRI osteoarthritis knee score) for the knee, HOAMS (hip osteoarthritis MRI scoring system) for the hip, and fixed-flexion radiography for measuring joint space width.

Arshed Quyyumi

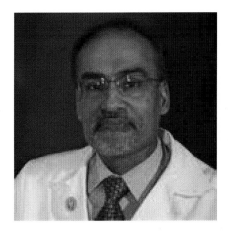

Cardiologist and director of Emory University's Clinical Cardiovascular Research Institute, Dr. Quyyumi is a high-profile medical researcher specializing in areas related to vascular biology, angiogenesis, progenitor cell biology, mechanisms of myocardial ischemia, and the role of genetic and environmental risks in vascular disease. He is an outspoken advocate of improving cardiology risk assessments and devoted to the improvement of cardiac care and a prolific author. His major impact on his field is demonstrated by more than 40,000 citations of his work in peer-reviewed scientific literature as well as an h-index of 102.

Nawal Nour

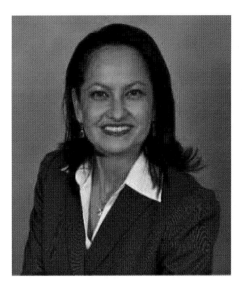

Dr. Nawal Nour is a preeminent public health and policy expert specializing in the eradication of female genital mutilation and the medical management of women who have experienced the event. Through her humanitarian work, she has been internationally recognized as a leading figure for the advocacy of women's public health awareness, garnering the prestigious MacArthur Fellowship in 2003.

Bulent Arslan

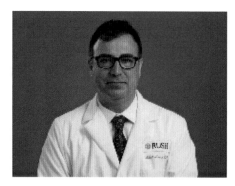

Dr. Bulent Arslan is an interventional radiologist and director of vascular and interventional radiology at Rush Medical Center in Chicago. He is lauded for his radically innovative new techniques in the treatment of aneurysms and critical limb ischemia (CLI). He is internationally recognized for his techniques and is a ubiquitous presenter/panelist at international meetings.

Mahmood Razavi

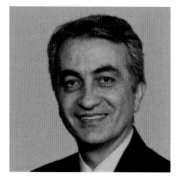

An expert in aneurysm and deep venous disease treatment and a prolific author of over 300 scientific publications, abstracts, and chapters, Dr. Razavi is the cofounder of six medical device companies with a total exit valuation of over $600 million. He holds thirty-nine US and international patents. In addition, Dr. Razavi is a current or past advisor to thirty-eight early-stage medical device companies with fourteen exit/IPOs to date and has served either on the board or as a strategic advisor to more than forty other medical companies.

He has been the recipient of several industry, institutional, and federal grants and has given over six hundred invited lectures at national and international scientific meetings. He has served as the global principal investigator in eight sponsored clinical trials and been the site principal investigator of another fifty multicenter studies. Dr. Razavi is currently the chief of Interventional Radiology Service as well as the Department of Clinical Trials and Research at St. Joseph Heart and Vascular Center in Orange, California. Dr. Razavi has pioneered many techniques for the crossing of lower extremity chronic total vascular occlusions. An internationally renowned expert in interventional radiology, he has been featured in more than 100 national and international radio, television, and press news articles and programs.

Syra Madad

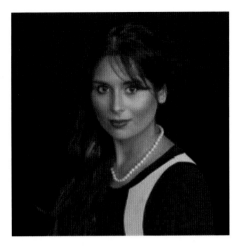

Syra Madad is an internationally recognized expert in public health—particularly the spread of infectious diseases—and is known as a pathogen preparedness pioneer. Working with her colleagues, she helped the Ebola Surge Team at the Texas Department of State Health Services deal with the first case of Ebola in the United States, which occurred at Texas Health Presbyterian Hospital in Dallas. For this work, she subsequently received an Ebola Response Appreciation Award. As of 2020, she is the senior director of the special pathogens program at New York City Health, one of the country's largest municipal healthcare delivery systems. A prominent educator and academic, Dr. Madad has taught numerous courses in such topics as advanced microbiology, biotechnology, and biosecurity, and she has received several recognitions involving the issues of special pathogen/disease control.

A dynamic author, editor, and speaker, she has written numerous peer-reviewed articles and presented her work at many conferences and other related events while being frequently quoted by many major news outlets. In 2020, Dr. Madad was featured for her work and diligence in the Netflix series Pandemic: How to Prevent an Outbreak, which concerned the control measures and science behind the spread of special and highly contagious diseases. She was also featured in the Discovery Channel documentary "The Vaccine: Conquering COVID." Dr. Madad is an inspiration to Muslims throughout the United States and the world for her passion and dedication in ensuring the public is protected from the dangers of pandemics.

Adah al-Mutairi

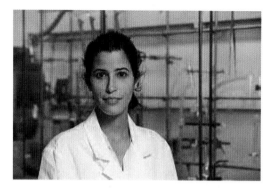

Adah al-Mutairi got her PhD from the University of California, Berkeley in chemical engineering in 2008, and went on to invent polymeric "nanocarriers" that can release drugs in response to certain physiological signals. Professor al-Mutairi is a world-renowned figure in the field of nanomedicine who developed particles for medical imaging, preventing blindness, and even to make an effective safer and faster way to do liposuction (removal of excess fat). She has thirteen patents to her name and was listed by Forbes as one of the top ten most influential engineers in the world and received the NIH Innovator Award for her work in 2009.

Salimuzzaman Siddiqui

Ajmaline is one of the most powerful drugs used to treat heart rhythm disturbances and therefore known as a Class 1A antiarrhythmic. In fact, the drug is used to diagnose the life-threatening heart condition Brugada syndrome, in a test called the Ajmaline Challenge. This drug, and its synthetic variant Prajmaline, is also used to treat other heart diseases. Renowned organic chemist Salimuzzaman Siddiqui discovered and synthesized Ajmaline in 1931 from the root and stem bark of a plant native to South Asia called Rauwolfia serpentina (Ajmaline was named after his legendary mentor Hakim Ajmal of Unami Medicine). Dr. Siddiqui went on to synthesize numerous drugs from the rauwolfia plant to treat mental and cardiovascular disorders as well as drugs to fight parasitic worms, bacteria, and viruses from the Neem tree. He received the Order of the British Empire in 1946 for this. He went on to found the Pakistan National Science Council, the Pakistan Academy of Sciences, and the Hussain Ebrahim Jamal Research Institute of Chemistry (known today as the International Center for Chemical and Biological Sciences).

Naweed Syed

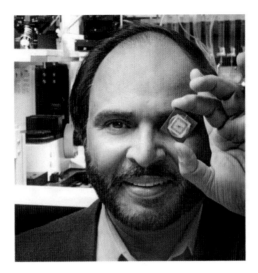

Dr. Syed made history with a scientific breakthrough, being the first to integrate brain cells to silicon microchips, known as the neurochip. Popularly known as bionics in science fiction (i.e., the popular TV series The Six Million Dollar Man), this invention brings this dream of integrating computers to the brain closer to reality. Dr. Syed's work with the neurochip will pave the way for bioengineers to "rebuild" people with sophisticated artificial limbs and even restoring memory loss or vision.

Hayat Sindi

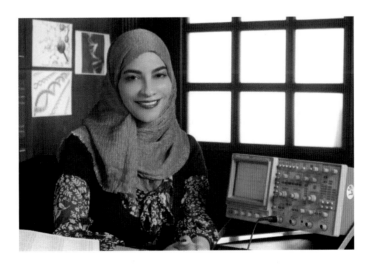

Hayat Sindi is an honored medical scientist who has developed an armament of low-cost, accessible, paper-based diagnostics designed to detect/diagnose disease with a single drop of body fluid (e.g., blood or urine) with her nonprofit company Diagnostics for All. Dr. Sindi has also contributed to work in the field of magnetic acoustic resonance assays for laboratory testing and is a leading advocate for empowering women scientists. In 2011 she founded i2institute, an organization that seeks to encourage science education and innovation among the youth.

Mohammed Mohiuddin

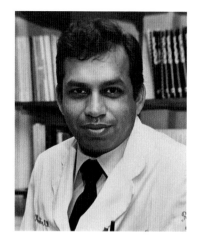

Dr. Mohiuddin is a trailblazing radiation oncologist who introduced a modernized version of GRID radiation therapy known as spatially fractionated radiation therapy (SFRT) more than thirty years ago with his megavoltage x-ray GRID SFRT. This innovative treatment (often described as working like magic) allows large, otherwise inoperable solid tumors to melt away by priming tumors with high and low doses of targeted radiation. It promises to be a safer and more effective treatment for certain previously untreatable advanced cancers than conventional radiation therapy, despite SFRT using only a fraction of the dose. It has opened up a new field of radiobiology. The story of SFRT and Dr. Mohiuddin is eloquently displayed in the dot decimal documentary Shine a Light: The History, Mystery, and Opportunity of GRID Therapy featuring his son, radiation oncologist Majid Mohiuddin. Additionally, Dr. Mohiuddin is an internationally recognized pioneer for a treatment approach to rectal cancer that would allow patients to avoid a colostomy bag. This approach produced a dramatic improvement in cure rates and is now the standard of care for locally advanced rectal cancer.

Hulusi Behçet

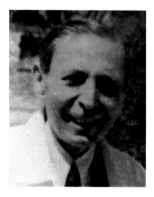

Dr. Hulusi Behçet was a dermatologist who made the groundbreaking discovery and classification of the eponymous skin disease Behçet syndrome. Behçet founded the department of dermatology and venereal diseases at the Istanbul University in 1933 and made seminal findings in 1937. This skin condition manifests with oral lesions, genital ulcers, ophthalmitis, and skin papules. The condition can affect multiple organs/systems and its discovery has been the source of many scientific inquiries/publications. Despite his outstanding achievements Behçet was dubbed "a scientist who was well known everywhere but in his country" by famous German pathologist Philip Schwartz.

Hasan Resat Sigindim

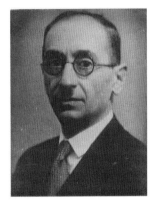

Dr. Sigindim, a Turkish physician, made important discoveries in the field of oncology. He was the first medical scientist to describe acute monocytic leukemia, after discovering unique properties of a syphilis patient diagnosed with acute leukemia.

Mehmet Esat Işık

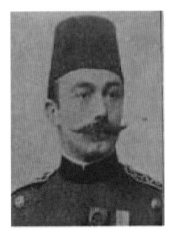

Dr. Mehmet Esat Işık, an ophthalmologist, revolutionized his field of medicine by making critical adjustments to the ophthalmoscope and creating the Essad ophthalmoscope, a device used for the diagnosis of certain ear and eye conditions. Dr. Mehmet Esat Işık was also a prolific poet, military officer, and politician. Additionally, he helped establish the Red Crescent Organization.

Ahmet Münir Sarpyener

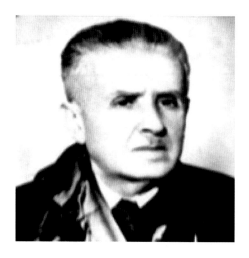

A Turkish spinal surgeon, Dr. Sarpyener helped define congenital spinal stenosis, a disorder displayed after birth in which the spinal canal is narrowed that progresses with age. He is considered a pioneer in his field for providing valuable contributions to the study/treatment of spina bifida and general spinal surgery techniques.

Abdel El-Mofty

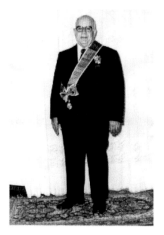

Psoralen is a substance from plants that can be activated by light. These were first used in combination with sunlight in ancient Egypt and India as far back as 2000–1200 BC to treat skin diseases. The ancients used these plant extracts by applying them directly to the skin or swallowing them to induce regeneration of skin coloration in a skin-whitening disease called vitiligo.

Abdel El-Mofty, an Egyptian dermatologist, was the first to report the use of a modern form of psoralen called 8-methoxy psoralen (8-MOP) with ultraviolet light for the treatment of vitiligo. Psoralens, usually in the form of 8-MOP, are now used with UV A light (called PUVA) to commonly treat skin diseases such as psoriasis (an autoimmune skin disease causing raised skin plaques), vitiligo and skin nodules of cutaneous T-cell lymphoma among thirty other skin diseases.

Ahmed Hani Weshahy

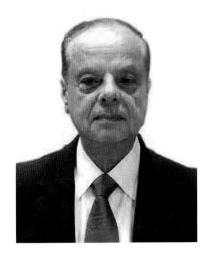

Keloids or abnormal scar tissue that builds up after an injury can be disfiguring and cause discomfort such as itching and pain. There was no ideal treatment if injecting the lesion with steroid or covering it with an occlusive silicone gel sheet failed. Previous surgical treatment resulted in high rate of recurrence and even worsening of the keloid. Even treatments including freezing it with liquid nitrogen (cryotherapy) from the surface were fraught with complications (infection, blistering, impaired healing, and loss of normal skin pigmentation) and could not reach the deeper layer to prevent recurrence. Dr. Weshahy devised a new technique using a hypodermic needle to deliver cryotherapy deeper and more precisely within the lesion without affecting the top layers, causing hypopigmentation and at the same time preventing recurrence. This technique, called intralesional cryotherapy, has been proven to be among the most effective treatment for keloids (reduction in volume by 63 percent at one year along with symptoms of itching and pain) and is now used to treat certain skin cancers.

Conclusion

Muslim innovation and contribution to the department of medicine is alive and well. The author humbly submits that there is no need to lament the loss of the golden age of Islamic medicine. The modern golden age of Islamic medicine is here and now. Unfortunately, many of the greatest contributors are actually refugees and pressured by Islamophobia to not identify themselves as Muslims. In fact, quite a few impactful physicians have declined recognition in this chapter. We should provide greater recognition from our communities through organizations such as IMANA and other Muslim societies. Recognition of achievement is necessary to counter Islamophobia and promote a more positive view of Islam and Muslims. If you speak with many scholars presented in this chapter, they are extremely humble despite the obstacles they have encountered. It is unfortunate that due to conditions in majority-Muslim countries, many of these great physicians and innovators are immigrants to the West and cannot perform their seminal contributions in their countries of origin.

Award/Honors Appendix

Abdul Mateen Ahmed

- President & CEO, New World Medical, Inc.
- Award of Excellence IMANA Ophthalmology 2016

Masood Akhtar

- Clinical Professor Medicine, University of Wisconsin School of Medicine and Public Health
- Director of Electrophysiology Research & Cardiovascular Continuing Medical Education Program, University of Wisconsin School of Medicine and Public Health
- Hypocrites Award for Excellence in Cardiovascular Disease Teaching, University of Florida-Miami School of Medicine, 1995
- Sir William Osler Award for Excellence in Cardiovascular Teaching, University of Miami
- Pioneer in Electrophysiology Award, by the Board of Trustees of the North American Society of Pacing and Electrophysiology, 1999
- Cardiovascular Researcher of the Year, American Heart Association (AHA), 1984
- President of the AHA Wisconsin Affiliate from 1996 to 1998

Adah Al-Mutairi

- Founder of eLux Medical Inc.
- Professor of Pharmaceutical Chemistry, University of California San Diego, Jacobs School of Engineering
- Director of the Center for Excellence in Nanomedicine and Engineering, Institute of Engineering in Medicine, University of California San Diego, Jacobs School of Engineering
- NIH Director New Innovator Award for NIH 2009
- phRMA Foundation Award 2009
- Thiema Chemistry Journal Award 2009
- Young Investigator Award, World Biomaterials Congress (Chengdu, China) 2012
- Young Investigator Award, American Chemical Society, 2014
- Royal Society of Chemistry 2014
- Kavli Fellow, US National Academy of Sciences 2016
- Forbes Top Ten Most Influential Woman Engineers 2021

Rozina Ali

- Cochrane Prize, St Thomas' Hospital
- Undergraduate Prize, Anatomical Society of Great Britain and Ireland
- International Microsurgery Fellowship, Chang Gung Memorial Hospital, Taiwan
- Cutlers' Surgical Fellowship, The Worshipful Company of Cutlers, London
- Healthcare Excellence Award
- Muslim Power 100, Parliamentary Review
- Pioneering Medical Woman Souvenir Edition Celebrating Centenary of the Medical Women's Federation (MWF)
- 'Best Aesthetic and Reconstructive Surgeon', Global Health & Pharma Magazine (GHP), 2019
- 'London's leading Aesthetic Surgeon', GHP Global Excellence awards, 2020

Syed Modasser Ali

- Executive Board Member WHO
- Director-General, Bangladesh Health Services, 2001
- Dean, Faculty of Postgraduate Medicine and Research, Dhaka University, 1998-2001
- Chairman of the Bangladesh Medical Research Council (1998-2003, 2017)
- Director/Professor Emeritus of the National Institute of Ophthalmology, Bangladesh (1997-2001)
- President of the Ophthalmic Society of Bangladesh
- Chairman, Governing Body, Dhaka City College
- Bangladesh National Personality Research Centre's Freedom Fighter Award
- WHO 50th Anniversary Primary Healthcare Development Award (1998)

- 20 Most Innovative Surgeons Alive Today (HAD.net, 2013)

Mohammed Abdul Aziz

- Senior Director, Clinical Research, Merck & Company's
- Barring an early death, Dr. Aziz would have certainly been highly honored and assuredly received the Nobel Prize in Medicine in 2015 that was awarded for successful demonstration of Ivermectin efficacy in treating African River Blindness.

Bulent Arslan

- Professor, Department of Diagnostic Radiology and Nuclear Medicine, RUSH Medical College
- Director, Vascular and Interventional Radiology, RUSH Medical College
- Top Doctor, Chicago Magazine, 2021, 2022
- Lifetime Centurion Reviewer Award, Journal of Vascular Interventional Radiology (JVIR), 2022
- Scientific Program Vice Chair, Society of Interventional Radiology, 2023

Hulusi Behçet

- Professor & Head of the Department of Dermatology and Venereal Diseases, Istanbul Unviersity
- TOBiTAK Scientific Award 1975
- Degree of Ordinarius, Dermatology Conference in Budapest 1935

Amman Bolia

- Consultant Vascular Radiologist, University Hospitals of Leicester, UK National Health Services (NHS) Trust
- Hospital Doctor of the Year, INNOVATION, UK, 1995
- Pioneers of Performance at Charing Cross 2016
- RW Günther Award for Excellence and Innovation by CIRSE 2012

Nadia Bukhari

Associate Professor, University College of London

Founder & Chief Operating Officer, Siha Health & Wellness

Director, Equity Pakistan

Global Lead Gender Equity, International Pharmaceutical Federation

Fellow of the Royal Pharmaceutical Society (RPS)

Chair and Organizer RPS Pre-registration Training Courses

Member of the National Pharmacy Board for England

Provost's Global Engagement Award

University College of London Global Pharmacy Ambassador

- Fellowship of the Higher Education Academy 2011
- Director of Education for PharmAesthetics UK

Mostafa El-Sayed

- Regents' Emeritus Professor, School of Chemistry & Biochemistry, Georgia Institute of Technology
- Julius Brown Chair, Department of Chemistry and Biochemistry, Georgia Institute of Technology
- Member of the President's National Medal of Science Committee 2014
- #17 in Thomson-Reuters Listing of the Top Chemists of the Past Decade 2011
- Ahmed Zewail Prize in Molecular Sciences 2009
- Glenn T. Seaborg Medal 2009
- Honorary Fellow of the Chinese Chemical Society 2009
- Medal of the Egyptian Republic, First Class 2009
- Inaugural Fellow of the American Chemical Society 2009
- Class of 1943 Distinguished Professor Award 2007
- President's National Medal of Science in Chemistry, National Sciences Foundation (NSF), 2007
- Langmuir Award of the American Chemical Society 2002
- Elected Fellow, American Association for the Advancement of Sciences 2000
- Elected Fellow, American Physical Society 2000
- King Faisal International Prize in the Sciences (Chemistry) 1990
- Elected Fellow of the American Academy of Arts and Sciences 1986
- Elected Member of the Third World Academy of Sciences 1984
- Alexander von Humboldt Senior Fellow 1982, 1982
- Elected Member of the US National Academy of Sciences 1980
- Alfred P. Sloan Fellow 1965–1971
- Fresenius National Award in Pure and Applied Chemistry 1967
- Guggenheim Foundation Fellow 1967–1968

Abdel El-Mofty

- Professor, Department of Dermatology, Cairo University
- Best Arab Doctor Award
- First Medical Doctor to Receive the Merit Distinction, Egypt
- First Medical Doctor to Receive the Republic Distinction, Egypt

Afshin Gangi

- Professor of Radiology, University Hospital Strasbourg, France
- Chairman of Radiology and Nuclear Medicine, University Hospital Strasbourg, France
- Chief, Interventional Radiology, University Hospital Strasbourg, France

- Lead in Oncological Interventional Radiology, Kings College London
- Professor of Interventional Oncology, Kings College London
- Deputy Chairman, European Conference on Interventional Oncology ECIO
- President, Cardiovascular and Interventional Radiology Society of Europe (CIRSE) 2019–2021
- Andreas Gruentzig Lecture CIRSE 2012
- Twice Elected as "Victoire de la Médecine" 2009 and 2010 France
- BSIR (British Society of Interventional Radiology) Honorary Fellow 2015
- Honorary Fellow German Society of Interventional Radiology (Ehrenmitglied DeGIR or Die Deutsche Gesellshaft für Interventionelle Radiologie und Minimal-Invasive Therapie) 2016
- Synergy Honors 2016

Mahmood Ghannoum

- Professor, Department of Dermatology, Case Western Reserve University, School of Medicine
- Professor, Department of Pathology, Case Western Reserve University, School of Medicine
- Director, Center for Medical Mycology, University Hospitals (Cleveland, OH)
- Chairman, Subcommittee on Antifungal Susceptibility Testing at the Clinical and Laboratory Standards Institute (CLSI)
- President of the Medical Mycological Society of the Americas
- Fellow of the Infectious Disease Society of America
- Freedom to Discover Award from Bristol-Myers Squibb (for his expertise in the field of fungal biofilms)
- Billy Cooper Award from the Mycological Societies of the Americas
- Cofounder of BIOHM Health, one of the leading consumer microbiome companies in the United States
- Founder of NTS Ventures, one of the leading microbiome and fungal clinical research organizations globally

Jafar Golzarian

- Professor of Radiology, University of Minnesota Medical School
- Vice Chair of Academic and Faculty Affairs, University of Minnesota Medical School
- Director, Division of Interventional Radiology & Vascular Imaging, University of Minnesota Medical School
- Co-director, Vascular Service Line, University of Minnesota Medical School
- Gold Medal, AVIR
- Gold Medal, Iranian Society of Radiology
- Honorary Member, Belgium Society of Radiology
- President, Association of the Chiefs of Interventional Radiology (2019)
- Minnesota Monthly Top Doctor (2018, 2021)

Ali Guermazi

- Professor of Radiology and Medicine
- Director of the Quantitative Imaging Center
- Assistant Dean of Diversity and Inclusion at Boston University School of Medicine
- Chief of Radiology at the VA Boston Healthcare System
- Editor-in-Chief of Skeletal Radiology
- President of the International Society of Osteoarthritis Imaging, 2019
- The Expert Radiologist to the International Olympics Committee
- Robert Coliez Award of the Scientific Exhibit, Paris 1995
- Scientific Exhibit Award: 82nd Scientific Assembly & Annual Meeting of the RSNA, Chicago 1996
- European Association of Radiology Exchange Program, Vienna 1997
- Scientific Exhibit Award: 10th European Congress of Radiology, Vienna 1997
- Visiting Scholar Program of the French Society of Radiology 1997
- Special Mention of the Scientific Exhibit, 46th French Congress of Radiology, Paris 1998
- Legion of Honor Awarded by the President of the Republic of Congo, Brazzaville 2000
- Radiological Society of North America Honored Educator Award 2012
- Abstract Awards in Clinical Science: 14th Annual EULAR Meeting, Madrid 2013
- Osteoarthritis Research Society International (ORSI) Clinical Research Award 2018
- RSNA Margulis Award for the Best Paper in 2022
- H-index of 111

Mahmood Hai

- President and Executive Director, The Surgical Institute of Michigan
- Senior Urologist, Affiliates Division of Comprehensive Urology, Division of Michigan Healthcare Professionals
- Fellowship of the International College of Surgeons 1994
- Institute for Social Policy and Understanding: Distinguished Award for Philanthropy 2007
- Honorary Fellowship of the Association of Surgeons of India 2009
- Dr. Edwin L. Thirlby Award: Best Presentation at the Annual Meeting of the North Central Section of the American Urological Association 2015
- Feature in the Muslim Americans for Progress: Impact Report of Muslim Contributions to Michigan 2017

Mark Humayan

- Professor of Ophthalmology, Keck School of Medicine, University of Southern California (USC)
- Cornelius J. Pings Chair in Biomedical Sciences, Keck School of Medicine, USC
- Director, Institute for Biomedical Therapeutics, Keck School of Medicine, USC

- Co-Director USC Roski Eye Institute
- Fellow IEEE
- H-index of 90
- Member of the US National Academy of Medicine
- Member of the US National Academy of Inventors
- Member of the US National Academy of Engineering
- U.S. News and World Report: Top 1% of Ophthalmologists
- Innovator of the Year, R & D Magazine, 2005
- Top 25 Inventions, Time Magazine, 2013
- National Medal of Technology and Innovation (United States' highest technological achievement) 2015
- IEEE Biomedical Engineering Award 2018
- IEEE Medal for Innovations in Healthcare Technology 2020

Muhammad Saiful Huq

- Professor Medical Physics, Radiation Oncology, University of Pittsburgh Medical Center (UPMC)
- Director of Medical Physics, Radiation Oncology, University of Pittsburgh Medical Center (UPMC)
- Founding Board Member, Journal of Biomedical Physics and Engineering Express, 2015
- Fellow, British Institute of Physics
- Fellow, American Association of Physicists in Medicine (AAPM)
- Farrington Daniels Award, AAPM
- Distinguished Service Award, American Board of Radiology 2010
- Distinguished Medical Physicist, Indo American Society of Medical Physicists 2010
- Vice Chair of the AAPM Science Council
- William D Coolidge Gold Medal, American Association of Physicists in Medicine (AAPM), 2023

Hamid Ikram

- Professor of Cardiology, St. George's Medical Centre (Christchurch, NZ)
- Recognized in the Queen's Birthday Honors 2017
- Officer of the New Zealand Order of Merit, For Significant Contributions to the Practice of Medicine in New Zealand, 2017

Mehmet Esat Işık

- Professor of Medicine, Imperial School of Medicine (Ottoman Empire)
- General Directorate of Health Affairs of the Ministry of Internal Affairs, Turkey

Malik Kahook

- Professor of Ophthalmology and The Slater Family Endowed Chair in Ophthalmology at the University of Colorado School of Medicine
- Vice Chair of Translational Research and serves as chief of the glaucoma service and director of the glaucoma fellowship at the University of Colorado Eye Center
- Editor of Essentials of Glaucoma Surgery, MIGS: Advances in Glaucoma Surgery and the seminal textbook of glaucoma Chandler and Grant's Glaucoma
- American Glaucoma Society Clinician Scientist Research Award 2007
- Inventor of the Year Award, University of Colorado, Denver 2009, 2010
- American Academy of Ophthalmology Achievement Award 2011
- Ludwig Von Sallmann Clinician-Scientist Award 2013
- #2 Top 40 under 40 Ophthalmologist List 2015
- The Ophthalmologist Top 100 Power List 2016

Muhammad Asim Khan

- Professor Emeritus of Medicine, Case Western Reserve University School of Medicine
- American College of Rheumatology's Distinguished Rheumatologist Award 2000
- Distinguished Rheumatologist Award from the American College of Rheumatology (ACR), 2002
- Elected Master of the American College of Physicians (MACP), 2003
- Elected Master of the American College of Rheumatology (MACR), 2009
- Inductee, Medical Hall of Honor of MetroHealth Medical Center, 2014
- Lifetime of Dedication and Devotion to People with Spondylitis Award from the Spondylitis Association of America (SAA), 1998
- First Recipient of the SAA's Greg Field Award, 2005
- Spondyloarthritis Research and Treatment Network (SPARTAN) Research Career Award, 2013
- Lifetime Achievement Award, Ohio Association of Rheumatology, 2015
- Teaching Excellence Award, MetroHealth Medical Center, 2006 & 2011
- Best Doctors in America, 2005-2012
- Distinguished Alumnus of Academic Excellence Award, King Edward Medical College Alumni Association of North America, 1998
- Pakistan Army Medical Corps Service Medal, 1966

Syra Madad

- Senior Director, System-wide Special Pathogens Program NYC Health + Hospitals
- Safety Lead of the Enhanced Investigations Unit of NYC Test and Trace Corp
- Fellow, Harvard Kennedy School Belfer Center for Science and International Affairs
- Special Pathogens Preparedness Pioneer Recognized as Emerging Leader

- J. V. Irons Award for Scientific Excellence
- Ebola Response Team Appreciation Award

Adel Mahmoud

- President, Vaccines Division, Merck & Co.
- President, International Society on Infectious Diseases
- Chair, Case Western Reserve University, School of Medicine, 1987-1998
- Bailey K. Ashford Medal 1983
- American Society of Tropical Medicine & Hygiene 1983
- Squibb Award of the Infectious Diseases Society of America 1984
- Consulted and Advised the NIH, the WHO, and Many Other Governmental Organizations

Ghaus Malik

- Executive Vice Chair, Department of Neurosurgery, Henry Ford Health Systems
- Community Service Award, Pakistan Association of America 1990
- Best Doctors in America 1990–Present
- Elected to Membership in the Society of Neurological Surgeons 1996
- John R. Davis Endowed Chair in Neurological Surgery 2004
- Henry Ford Medical Association's Distinguished Career Award 2006
- Fred Whitehouse Award 2006
- Lifetime Achievement Award, Association of Pakistani Physicians of North America 2008
- Malik Lectureship in Neurosurgery 2011
- APPNA Pioneers Award, Association of Pakistani Physicians of North America, Michigan 2011
- Senior Staff Teaching Award 2013–2014
- Senior Staff Teaching Award 2014–2015
- Walter E. Dandy Medal Recipient 2015
- Lifetime Achievement Award Association of Pakistani Physician of North America Michigan Chapter 2017
- Henry Ford West Bloomfield Hospital Service Award 2017
- Wayne County Medical Society Celebration of Fifty Years in Medicine 1968–2018
- Gold Pin Award by Michigan State Medical Society for Fifty years of Medical Service 2018
- Distinguished Alumni Award 2020
- Albert Nelson Marquis Lifetime Achievement Award 2022

Kazi Mobin-Uddin

- Professor Cardiothoracic Surgery, Ohio State College of Medicine, The Ohio State University
- Device Named by Newsweek as the "Umbrella of Life"

- Star of Achievement (SITARA – I – IMTIAZ) Government of Pakistan (Highest Civilian Achievement) 1970

Frederick Akbar Mohamed

- Pupil's Physical Society Prize
- Royal College of Surgeons 1872
- Elected Fellow, Royal College of Physicians, 1880

Mohammed Mohiuddin

- Fellow of American College of Radiology
- Fellow of American Society for Radiation Oncology
- Fellow of American College of Radiation Oncology

Muhammed Mansour Mohiuddin

- Professor of Surgery, University of Maryland School of Medicine
- Chief of transplantation section of Cardiothoracic Surgery Research Program and Senior Scientist at the National Heart Lung and Blood Institute of the National Institutes of Health
- Director, Cardiac Xenotransplantation Program at University of Maryland
- Named by Nature journal as one of the top 10 people who helped shaped science in 2022
- Awarded a honorary degree of Doctorate in Science from Dow University of Health Sciences, Karachi, Pakistan
- National Research Service Award / NIH
- Recognition by Maryland State Legislature for Outstanding Medical Research
- APPNA Award for Professional Excellence
- DOGANA Award for Groundbreaking, Unparalleled and Nobel Prize Worthy Research in Organ Transplantation
- DOGANA Lifetime Achievement Award 2023 – Dallas, Texas

Amir Mortajeme

- Founder & Director, Midwest Vascular Institute of Illinois
- Chairman of Department of Radiology at St. Anne's Hospital
- Lifetime Recognition Award, Chicago Endovascular Conference
- Fellow of the Society for Interventional Radiology
- Physicians Recognition Award, American Medical Association

Tofigh Mussivand

- Chair & Director, Cardiovascular Devices Research Laboratory, University of Ottawa Heart Institute

- Chair of the Medical Devices Program, University of Ottawa
- Professor of Surgery, University of Ottawa
- Professor of Engineering, School of Information Technology and Engineering, University of Ottawa
- Professor, Mechanical and Aerospace Engineering, Carleton University
- Established, Medical Devices Commercialization Centre (Networks of Centres of Excellence of Canada)
- Knowledge Translation Award, Canadian Institute of Health Research (CIHR) (2010)
- CIHR Health Researcher of the Year 2010
- Ottawa Life Sciences Council Annual Achievement Awards 1997
- Fellow of the Royal Society of Canada (Highest Scholarly Honor in Canada)
- Honorary Member of the Iranian Academy of Medical Sciences
- Queen Elizabeth II Diamond Jubilee Medal, 2013
- John Foerster Distinguished Lecturer Award, Institute of Cardiovascular Sciences, 2010
- Lifetime Achievement Award, Regional Innovation, National Research Council of Canada, 2001
- Synergy Award, Natural Sciences and Engineering Research Council of Canada and the Conference Board of Canada, 2000
- Ottawa Life Sciences Entrepreneurial Award, 1999
- President's Award, Ottawa Centre for Research and Innovation (OCRI), 1999
- Brazilian Cardiac Surgeons Award, Brazilian Society of Cardiovascular Surgery (BCS), 1998
- MEDEC Award for Medical Achievement, Canadian Medical Device Industry Association, 1998
- Applied Research Award, Ottawa Life Sciences Council (1997)
- Hippocratic Plaque, World Society of Cardio-Thoracic Surgeons, 2008
- Nominated, Michael Smith Award for Excellence, 1998
- Notable Mention, "Inventing Canada", Medical Wonders: The HeartSaver, 1997

Jihad Mustapha

- Nicknamed the 'Leg Saver'
- President, CEO & Director of Endovascular Interventions, Advanced Cardiac & Vascular Centers
- Platinum Level Reviewer 2018. Journal of Invasive Cardiology
- Innovation Health Hero Award. West Michigan Alliance for Health 2013
- West Michigan Health Innovation Hero Presented by Alliance for Health 2013
- Founder & Director of the AMPutation Prevention Symposium (AMP)
- Founding Board Member of the CLI Global Society
- America's Vascular Team of the Year 2023 (CLI-Courses Global Vascular Awards)

Alexander Norbash

- Chair & Professor, Radiology, University of California, San Diego (UCSD) Health
- Chair & Professor, Radiology, Boston University from 2004 to 2015

- Adjunct Professor, Neurosurgery, UCSD
- Associate Vice Chancellor, Diversity, Equity and Inclusion, UCSD
- Co-Directors, Center for Cardiovascular Biomedical Imaging (CCBI), UCSD
- Director, Diagnostic and Interventional Neuroradiology Service, Brigham and Women's Hospital
- Founder, Interventional Neuroradiology and Endovascular Neurosurgical Practices, Brigham and Women's Hospital
- President of the Society of Chairs of Academic Radiology, 2018-2020
- President of the New England Roentgen Ray Society 2007–2008
- President of the Massachusetts Radiological Society 2015–2016
- Board Member of the Society for Chairs of Academic Radiology Departments
- Board Member of the American College of Radiology
- Board Member American Roentgen Ray Society
- Member of the American College of Radiology's Board of Chancellors
- "Top Doctor" in Radiology by Boston Magazine
- "America's Top Doctors", Castle Connolly Medical
- UMKC (University of Missouri, Kansas City) Alumnus of the Year 2020

Nawal Nour

- Chair, Department of Obstetrics and Gynecology, Brigham and Women's Hospital
- Established, African Women's Health Center, 1999
- Kate Macy Ladd Professorship, Obstetrics and Gynecology, Harvard Medical School
- Commonwealth Fund/Harvard University Fellowship in Health Policy
- Director of Obstetric Ambulatory Practice at the Harvard-Affiliated Brigham and Women's Hospital
- MacArthur Fellows Program 2003
- Reede Scholar 1998–1999
- AMWA's Lila A. Wallis Women's Health Award 2012
- Forbes' 40 Women to Watch, 2017
- Initialing, Philosopher's Legacy

Ahmed Okasha

- Professor & Founder, Okasha Institute of Psychiatry
- Director, Collaborating Center for Training & Research in Mental Health, WHO
- Faculty of Medicine, Ain Shams University, Egypt
- President of the World Psychiatric Association (WPA) 2002–2005
- President of the Egyptian Society of Biological Psychiatry
- President of the World Federation of Societies of Biological Psychiatry (WFSBP)
- Chairman of WPA Review Committee 2008–2011
- Chairman of WPA Ethics' Committee 1993–2002

- Chairman, Scientific Committee of Egyptian Board of Psychiatry
- Chairman, Egyptian Board of Child & Adolescent Psychiatry
- Chairman, Egyptian Board of Addiction Psychiatry
- Golden Medal of International Association for Child and Adolescent Psychiatry and Allied Professions' (ICAPAP) 2004
- State Prize in Creativity in Medicine, Egyptian Academy of Science, 2000
- Honorary Fellowship of the American College of Psychiatrists 2002
- Presidential Commendation of American Psychiatric Association (APA), 2006
- State Merit Award in Medical Sciences, Egyptian Academy of Science, 2007
- El Nil Merit Award in Medical Sciences 2010
- Awarded Kraeplin – Alzheimer Medal, Munich University, 2012
- Medal of Science and Arts of the First Degree, Egyptian Academy of Science, 2013
- Honorary Fellow of WPA 2005
- Honorary Doctorate in Science from Ain Shams University, Cairo 2019
- Member of National Mental Health Council
- Member of Supreme Council of Culture
- Member of Supreme Council of Health
- Member of National Council Addressing Fundamentalism and Terrorism
- Honorary President of the Arab Federation of Psychiatrists
- Honorary Doctorates & Fellowships, Numerous Universities and Psychiatric Associations

Ayub Ommaya

- Chief of Neurosurgery, National Institute of Neurological Diseases (NINDS), NIH
- Chair, Neurosurgery, George Washington University
- Chief Medical Adviser, US National Highway Traffic Safety Administration
- Rhodes Scholarship Recipient
- Creator, National Center for Injury Prevention and Control, Center for Disease Controls
- Founding Member, Association of Physicians of Pakistani Descent of North America (APPNA)
- Honorary Physician to the President of Pakistan 1983–1988
- Star of Achievement (SITARA – I – IMTIAZ) Government of Pakistan (Highest Civilian Achievement) 1982
- Considered Nobel-Prize Winning Prospect, by Nobel Laureate Barry Blumberg, MD

Mehmet Oz

- Vice Chair & Professor Emeritus, Surgery, Vagelos College of Physicians & Surgeons, Columbia University
- Director, Cardiovascular Institute & Complementary Medicine Program, New York Presbyterian Hospital

- Lois Pope LIFE International Research Award, Leonard M. Miller School of Medicine, University of Miami, 2008
- Nine Emmy Awards for Informative/Outstanding Talk Shows
- Hollywood Star Recipient
- New York Times "Bestseller's List"
- Named 'Global Leader of Tomorrow', World Economic Forum, 2004
- Doctor of the Year by Hippocrates Magazine
- "100 Most Influential People", Time Magazine, 2008
- National Magazine Award for Personal Service, 2009
- Co-Creator, Dr. Oz The Good Life Magazine

Resad Pazic

- Professor, Obstetrics & Gynecology, Department of OB/GYN & Women's Health, University of Louisville
- Director, Fellowship in Minimally Invasive Gynecologic Surgery (MIGS), Department of OB/GYN & Women's Health, University of Louisville
- John Stegee Mentorship Award, American Association of Gynecological Laproscopists (AAGL), 2022
- Honorary Chair of 51st Annual AAGL Global Congress, 2020
- President, International Society of Gynecologic Endoscopy (ISGE), 2019-2021
- President, AAGL, 2009
- President, Fellowship Board of the AAGL/SRS sponsored Fellowship in Endoscopy and Minimally Invasive Surgery, 2010
- Awarded "Best Doctors in America" for 2005-2006, 2007-2008, 2009-2010, 2014-2018
- Awarded Top Surgeons in Louisville 2010-2013

Arshad Quadri

- Cardiothoracic surgery specialist in West Hartford, CT
- Chairman, CMO, CardiAQ Valve Technologies
- Prize-Winning Paper (Fifth Annual Vascular Symposium) 1991
- Association of Physicians of Pakistani Descent of North America, Scientific Achievement Award 2017

Arshed Quyyumi

- Professor of Medicine, Cardiology, Emory University School of Medicine
- Director, Emory Clinical Cardiovascular Institute
- R. Wayne Alexander Excellence in Research Accomplishment Award at the Emory University Department of Medicine 2016
- MRCP, Royal College of Physicians 1979

Shahbuddin Rahimtoola

- 'Cardiologist of the World' & 'Father of Research', European Heart Journal, 2013
- Distinguished Professor at the Keck School of Medicine, University of Southern California
- George C. Griffith Professor of Cardiology, University of Southern California (USC)
- Chief, Cardiology, USC
- Chairman, Council on Clinical Cardiology, American Heart Association (AHA)
- Trustee, American College of Cardiology (ACC)
- Citations for International Service and Outstanding Service, American Heart Association (AHA), 1985
- Editor-in-Chief, Current Topics in Cardiology
- Sir William Osler Award, University of Miami
- Gifted Teacher Award, American College of Cardiology (ACC), 1986
- Award of Merit and Special Recognition, AHA, 1985
- James B. Herrick Award, AHA, 1989
- Melvin L. Marcus Memorial Award, International Society of Heart Failure, 1996
- Distinguished Alumnus Award from the Mayo Clinic Foundation 1998
- Mayo Clinic's All-Time Top Fifty Practitioners
- Silver Medal Denolin from the European Society of Cardiology
- Federal Drug Administration's Harvey W. Wiley Medal
- Sheikh Hamdan Award for Medical Science, UAE Government, 2000
- Distinguished Scientist Award, ACC, 2001
- Honorary Doctor of Science, University of Karachi, 2002
- Gold Medal, European Society of Cardiology, 2009
- Lifetime Achievement, ACC, 2013
- 'Distinguished Fellowship' Award, World Congress of International Academy of Cardiology, 2016

Azra Raza

- Chan Soon-Shiong Professor, Medicine, Vagelos College of Physicians & Surgeons, Columbia University
- Clinical Director, The Evans Foundation Myelodysplastic Syndrome Center, Vagelos College of Physicians & Surgeons, Columbia University
- Member, Founder Group, with designing Breakthrough Developments in Science and Technology with President Clinton designing Breakthrough Developments in Science and Technology and with VP Joe Biden for the Cancer Moonshot initiative
- First Lifetime Achievement Award, APPNA
- Award in Academic Excellence from Dogana 2007, 2010
- Woman of the Year Award from Safeer e Pakistan, California
- Hope Award in Cancer Research 2012

- '100 Women Who Matter' by Newsweek Pakistan March 2012

Fadi Saab

- Judge, Clinical Research Day, Metro Health – University of Michigan Health 2012–Present
- Co-Founder & COO, Advanced Cardiac and Vascular Amputation Prevention Centers (ACV)
- Chief Interventional Cardiology Fellow. Baystate Medical Center; Springfield, MA 2010–2011
- Chief General Cardiology Fellow. Baystate Medical Center 2009–2010
- Cardiovascular Fellow of the Year Award. Baystate Medical Center 2008–2009
- Life & Limb Saving Award, Outpatient Endovascular & Interventional Society (OEIS), 2022
- America's Vascular Team of the Year 2023 (CLI-Courses Global Vascular Awards)

Moncef Saloui

- Professor, Immunology, University of Mons, Belgium
- Chair, Board of Directors, Galvani Bioelectronics
- Chairman, Vaccines, GlaxoSmithKline (GSK)
- Chairman, Global Research & Development, GSK PLC
- Head, Operation Warp Speed: Project Dedicated to Finding the COVID-19 Vaccine 2020
- National Academies of Sciences, Engineering, and Medicine, Forum on Medical and Public Health Preparedness for Disasters and Emergencies, Member
- Human Vaccines Project, Board Member 2018
- Honorary Doctor of Science, Gettysburg College 2017
- 25 Most influential People in Biopharma Today by Fierce Biotech 2012
- World's 50 Greatest Leaders by Fortune 2016
- "World's Top 100 Medicine Makers" by the Medicine Maker 2018
- Great Immigrants Honoree, Carnegie Corporation of New York, 2023
- Member, Board of Directors, International AIDS Vaccine Initiative
- Mosquitrix (first malaria vaccine), Cervarix (prevent cervical cancer), Ebola, Rotarix (prevention of diarrhea in children), Synflorix (pneumococcal disease)
- "Arguably the world's most experienced and successful vaccine developer." Alex Azar, Secretary of Health and Human Services

Madjid Samii

- Chairman, Neurosurgery, Hannover School of Medicine, Germany
- Honorary President of World Federation of Neurosurgical Societies
- President of the International Neuroscience Institute (INI) at Otto von Guericke University
- President of the International Society for Neurosurgery
- President of the China INI at Capital University in Beijing

- President of the Neurobionic Foundation
- Elected as the founding president of MASCIN – "Madjid Samii Congress of International Neurosurgeons" in 2003
- President of the Board of Trustees of AWD Children's Assistance Foundation
- Director emeritus of the Neurosurgical Clinic, Nordstadt Hospital in Hannover
- Honorary President of the World Federation of Neurosurgical Societies (WFNS)
- Honorary President of the World Federation of Neurosurgical Societies Endowment/Foundation (WFNS)
- Honorary President of the German Society of Skull Base Surgery
- Honorary President of CURAC - German Society of Computer and Robot-Assisted Surgery
- Award of the „Aristoteles Gold Medal" by the University of Thessaloniki, Greece, June 1998
- Rudolf Frey Award, 2000
- Paul C. Bucy Award, 2003
- Avicenna Award, 2006
- INC Award, 2006
- Iranian Science and Culture Hall of Fame 2006
- World Physician, City of Hannover, Germany, 2007
- Friendship Award, People's Republic of China, 2007
- Neurosurgical Society of America Medal Recipient 2010
- Leibniz-Ring-Hannover Prize 2013
- Neurosurgeon of the Year, World Neurosurgery Journal 2013
- Leibniz-Ring-Hannover Award, 2013
- World Intellectual Property Organization (WIPO) Award, 2014
- World Top Neurosurgeon, 2014
- Golden Neuron Award, 2014
- Kharazmi International Award, 2014
- Nobel medal by the professor of neurosurgical department at Karolinska Institute
- Member of the nobel prize committee, Stockholm, Sweden, 22-Sep-1987
- Obrador Medal, Madrid, Spain, 1989
- Jamieson Medal, Australia, 1991
- Sir Charles Balance Medal, London, England, 1997
- Honorary Doctorates & Fellowship from Numerous Countries

Ugur Sahin

- Founder and CEO of BioNTech
- Professor for Translational Oncology and Immunology at University Medical Center Mainz
- Full Professor (W3) in Translational Oncology & Immunology at Johannes Gutenberg University in Mainz, Germany

- Chairman of the Scientific Management Board of the Helmholtz Institute for Translational Oncology (HI-TRON), also in Mainz, Germany
- Initiated and oversaw "Project Lightspeed," the historic development of the first mRNA vaccine for COVID-19
- Vincenz Czerny Prize of the German Society of Hematology and Oncology (DGHO) 1995
- Merit Award of the American Society of Clinical Oncology 1995
- Calogero Paglierello Research Award 1997
- Georges Köhler Prize of the German Society of Immunology 2005
- GO-Bio Prize of the Federal Ministry of Education and Research 2006, 2010
- BMBF Spitzencluster Award for TRON projects as part of CI3-Regional Cluster for Individualized Immune Intervention 2012
- ERC Advanced Grant in Life Sciences 2017–2018
- Mustafa Prize 2019
- German Cancer Award 2019
- National German Sustainability Award 2020
- Financial Times Person of the Year 2020
- Knight Commander's Cross of the Order of Merit of the Federal Republic of Germany 2012
- Princess of Asturias Award in the category "Scientific Research" 2021

Aziz Sancar

- Sarah Graham Kenan Professor of Biochemistry and Biophysics, UNC School of Medicine
- Adjunct Appointment in Biology
- Nobel Prize in Chemistry 2015
- Turkish Koç Award 2007
- University of Texas at Dallas Distinguished Alumni Award 2009
- TWESCO International Turkish Academy – Gold Medal at UN 2016
- Bert and Natalie Vallee Award 2016
- National Academy of Medicine 2016
- Member Turkish Academy of Sciences 2006
- Member American Academy of Arts and Sciences 2004
- Member National Academy of Sciences, United States 2005
- Member American Society for Biochemistry & Molecular Biology
- Distinguished Alumni Award (Univ. of Texas at Dallas) 2009
- O. Max Gardner Award (highest honor by University of North Carolina Board of Governors) 2016
- Carnegie Corporation's Immigrant of the Year 2016
- North Carolina Award (the highest civilian honor given by the state) 2016
- National Academy of Medicine 2016
- Lifetime Achievement Award (Univ. of Texas at Dallas) 2018

- Hyman L. Battle Distinguished Cancer Research Award 2019
- Honorary Doctorates from Turkey, Azerbaijan, Kazakhstan, Kyrgyzstan, Uzbekistan, Peru 2006-2022

Husain Sattar

- Professor of Pathology University of Chicago's Pritzker School of Medicine
- Associate Director of the clinical pathophysiology and therapeutics course at the Pritzker School of Medicine
- Outstanding Basic Science Teaching Award
- Favorite Faculty Award, University of Chicago School of Medicine

Khalid Shah

- Vice Chair of Research for the Department of Neurosurgery at BWH
- Professor at Harvard Medical School.
- Director, The Center for Stem and Translational Immunotherapy
- Director, Joint Center of Excellence in Biomedicine
- Principal Faculty at Harvard Stem Cell Institute in Boston.
- Research Fellow Award, American Cancer Society
- Innovation Awards from James McDonnell Foundation, ABTA, Goldhirsh Foundation and American Association of Radiology
- Distinguished Research Award from the Academy of Radiology
- Department of Defence Idea and Impact Award
- Young Investigator Award, Alliance for Cancer Gene Therapy (ACGT)
- Young Mentor Award from Harvard University

Mehdi Shishehbor

- President of University Hospitals Harrington Heart and Vascular Institute where he is the Angela and James Hambrick Master Clinician in Innovation
- Professor, Case Western Reserve University School of Medicine
- Director of the Cardiovascular Interventional Center, and co-director of the Vascular Center for UH Harrington Heart & Vascular Institute
- CMO of Inquis Medical
- Co-chair of the PVD Council for Society for Cardiovascular Angiography
- Interventions (SCAI)
- Member of PVD council for the American College of Cardiology (ACC)
- Carol and Arthur F. Anton Leadership Fellowship Program Award 2018
- Recognized by University Hospitals as a Distinguished Physician 2020
- National Institutes of Health scholar

- Thomas J. Linnemeier Spirit of Interventional Cardiology Young Investigator Award 2008
- VIVA/LINC Young Leader's Award in Vascular 2009
- Chair of the Masters' Approach to Critical Limb Ischemia (MAC) Symposium in 2016
- Co-Founder of Cardiovascular Innovations Annual Meeting and Foundation
- Crain's Notable Immigrant Leader Award 2022

Teepu Siddique

- Les Turner ALS Foundation/Herbert C. Wenske Foundation Professor at the Feinberg School of Medicine
- Chief Scientific Officer Novel Therapies, LLC
- American Academy of Neurology Sheila Essey Award
- Rattigan Medal from the University of the Punjab
- Hope through Caring Award from the Les Turner ALS Foundation
- Forbes Norris Award from the International Alliance of ALS/MND Associations
- First Abbott Laboratories Susan and Duane Burnham Research Professor
- Fogarty International Scholar at the National Institute for Neurologic Diseases and Stroke

Salimuzzaman Siddiqui

- Professor of Chemistry, University of Karachi
- Order of the British Empire 1946
- Foundation Fellow, Pakistan Academy of Sciences 1953
- D. Med. Honoris causa, Frankfurt University 1958
- Hilal-e-Imtiaz (Crescent of Excellence), Government of Pakistan 1980
- President Pan-Indian Ocean Science Association 1960
- President of Pakistan's Pride of Performance Medal 1966
- Sitara-e-Imtiaz (Star of Excellence), Government of Pakistan 1962
- Fellow of the Royal Society 1961
- Tamgha-e-Pakistan (Medal of Pakistan) 1958
- Third World Academy of Sciences – TWAS Prize 1985
- Founded the Hussain Ebrahim Jamal Research Institute of Chemistry
- Gold Medal of the Soviet Academy of Sciences

Alam Nisar Syed

- Medical Director for Long Beach Memorial Hospital
- Celebration of Life Medical Honoree Award from the American Cancer Society 2017
- Founder American Brachytherapy Society
- Program director for the National Healthcare Group Medical Oncology Residency Program

- Founder Journal of Brachytherapy International

Naweed Syed

- Professor at the Cumming School of Medicine, University of Calgary
- Research Director HBI at the Cumming School of Medicine, University of Calgary
- Postdoctoral Program Director – Cumming School of Medicine, University of Calgary
- Office of the Vice President (Research) Cumming School of Medicine, University of Calgary
- Parker B. Francis Fellowship 1992
- Alfred P. Sloan Fellowship
- Alberta Heritage Foundation for Medical Research Scholarship Medical Scientist Awards
- Canadian Institutes for Health Research (CIHR) Investigator Award
- Outstanding Collaboration Award, Schulich School of Engineering 2012
- Canadians for Global Care Award of Recognition 2015
- Fellowship from the Royal Society of Edinburgh, UK
- Tamgha e Imtiaz (Medal of Excellence) 2017
- Senate of Canada 150 Medal 2017
- Outstanding Scientist Award from the Asian Community in Toronto 2004
- Canadian Sensation Award from South Asian Media Express Network 2012
- Distinguished Achievement Award for Outstanding Contributions to Biomedical Research by Pakistan-Canada Association 2012

Hayat Sindi

- Saudi Arabian medical scientist
- One of the first female members of the Consultative Assembly of Saudi Arabia
- Makkah Al-Mukaramah' Prize for Scientific Innovation, Saudi Arabia 2010
- Emerging Explorer, National Geographic Society 2011
- 150 Women Who Shake the World, Newsweek 2012
- UNESCO Goodwill Ambassador 2012
- Global Citizens Award, Clinton Foundation 2014
- Member of the Scientific Advisory Board, UN, 2013
- Listed as one of BBC's 100 Women 2018
- Ranked by Arabian Business as the 19th most influential Arab in the world and the 9th most influential Arab woman

Ozlem Tureci

- Co-founded the biotechnology company BioNTech
- Chief Medical Officer BioNTech

- Professor of Personalized Immunotherapy at the Helmholtz Institute for Translational Oncology (HI-TRON) and Johannes Gutenberg University Mainz
- Vincenz Czerny Prize of the German Society of Hematology and Oncology (DGHO) 1995
- Calogero Paglierello Research Award 1997
- Georges Köhler Prize of the German Society of Immunology 2005
- National German Sustainability Award 2020
- Financial Times Person of the Year (with Uğur Şahin) 2020
- Axel Springer Award (with Uğur Şahin) 2021
- Order of Merit of the Federal Republic of Germany 2021
- Princess of Asturias Award in the category "Technical and Scientific Research" (with Uğur Şahin and five others 2021

Muhammad Basharat Yunus

- Professor of Medicine at the University of Illinois College of Medicine
- Father of Modern View of Fibromyalgia
- Physician Recognition Award, University of Illinois College of Medicine at Peoria 1996
- Distinguished Alumni Award (Research), Chittagong Medical College Bangladesh 2007
- Annual Celebration of Excellence Award, University of Illinois College of Medicine at Peoria 2009–2015
- Raymond B. Allen (Golden Apple) Instructorship Award

Salim Yusuf

- Marion W. Burke Chair in Cardiovascular Disease at McMaster University Medical School
- President of the World Congress of Cardiology 2015 and 2016
- Initiated the Emerging Leaders Program of the World Congress of Cardiology
- Officer in the Order of Canada 2013
- Canada Gairdner Wightman Award
- Canadian Medical Hall of Fame
- President of the World Heart Federation
- He was the world's second-most cited cardiology researcher 2011
- He was the most-cited scientist in the world in cardiology 2020
- Awarded McLaughlin medal of the Royal Society of Canada 2020
- Awarded Killam prize 2022

Sherif Zaki

- Chief Pathologist, CDC
- Founder/Chief Infectious Disease Pathology Branch, CDC

- 9x Distinguished Service Award, U.S. Health and Human Services Secretary (Department's highest honor)
- Charles C. Shepard Science Award 2004, 2007, 2017

Elias Zerhouni

- Knight of the Légion d'Honneur (French National Order of the Legion of Honor)
- Gold Medal from the American Roentgen Ray Society
- Paul Lauterbur Awards for MRI Research
- Presidential Award of the European Congress of Radiology
- Senior Fellow of the Bill and Melinda Gates Foundation
- Member of the Institute of Medicine of the US National Academy of Sciences 2000
- French Academy of Medicine 2010
- Member National Academy of Medicine 2000
- Member US National Academy of Engineering
- Board Member Lasker Foundation, Research America and NIH Foundation

Huda Zoghbi

- Professor, Departments of Molecular and Human Genetics, Neuroscience and Neurology at the Baylor College of Medicine.
- Jan and Dan Duncan Neurological Research Institute
- Editor of the Annual Review of Neuroscience, 2018
- Watanabe Prize, Translational Research, Clinical and Translational Sciences Institute (CTSI), 2023
- Kavli Prize Laureate, Neuroscience, Norwegian Academy of Sciences, 2022
- Victor A. McKusick Leadership Award, American Society of Human Genetics 2019
- Member American Academy of Arts and Sciences 2018
- Ross Prize in Molecular Medicine 2018
- National Order of the Cedar, Lebanon 2018
- Breakthrough Prize in Life Sciences 2017
- Canada Gairdner International Award 2017
- Jessie Stevenson Kovalenko Medal 2016
- Shaw Prize in Life Science and Medicine 2016
- Mechthild Esser Nemmers Prize in Medical Science, Northwestern University 2015
- Vanderbilt Prize in Biomedical Science, Vanderbilt University School of Medicine 2015
- Javits Neuroscience Investigator Award, National Institute of Neurological Disorders and Stroke (NINDS), National Institutes of Health 2015
- Mortimer D. Sackler, M.D. Prize for Distinguished Achievement in Developmental Psychobiology, Weill Cornell Medicine and Columbia University College of Physicians and Surgeons 2015
- Honorary Doctor of Medical Sciences, Yale University 2014

- March of Dimes Prize in Developmental Biology 2014
- Edward M. Scolnick Prize in Neuroscience, McGovern Institute for Brain Research, Massachusetts Institute of Technology 2014
- Dickson Prize in Medicine, University of Pittsburgh 2013
- Pearl Meister Greengard Prize, Rockefeller University 2013
- Gruber Prize in Neuroscience 2011
- Vita and Lee Lyman Dewey Tuttle Brookwood Legacy Award for Excellence and Partnership in Medicine, Brookwood Community 2011
- International Rett Syndrome Foundation's Circle of Angels Research Award 2009
- Vilcek Prize for Biomedical Research, Vilcek Foundation 2009
- Marion Spencer Fay Award, Drexel University College of Medicine 2009
- Cathedra Laboris, University of Monterrey 2009
- Honorary Doctor of Science, Meharry Medical College 2008
- Texas Women's Hall of Fame 2008
- Perl-UNC Neuroscience Prize 2007
- Robert J. and Claire Pasarow Foundation Award in Neuropsychiatry Research 2007
- Member of the National Academy of Sciences 2004
- Neuronal Plasticity Prize, Ipsen Foundation 2004
- Marta Philipson Award in Pediatrics, Philipson Foundation for Research 2004
- Fellow of the American Association for the Advancement of Science 2002
- Bernard Sachs Award, Society for Pediatric Research 2001
- Member of the National Academy of Medicine formerly the Institute of Medicine 2000
- Sidney Carter Award, American Academy of Neurology 1998
- Javits Award, NINDS, National Institutes of Health 1998
- E. Mead Johnson Award, Society of Pediatric Research 1996
- Kilby International Award 1995

References

1. Torres, Vicki. "Southern California Enterprise: Seeing Is Believing: Rancho Cucamonga Firm's Glaucoma Valve Looks Like a Hit." LA Times. May 8, 1995.

2. "Onchocerciasis (River Blindness): Disease Information." World Health Organization. November 20, 2018. www.who.int/blindness/partnerships/onchocerciasis_disease_information/en.

3. Hoque, Leedy. "In Memory of Dr. Mohammed Abdul Aziz, a Trailblazer in Medicine." The Daily Star. November 30, 2015. www.thedailystar.net/op-ed/trailblazer-medicine-179983.

4. Ozkan, J., "Prof. Shahbudin H. Rahimtoola MB, FRCP, MACC, MACP, FESC, DSc (Hon) has been described as a cardiologist of the world and the father of research and clinical practice in myocardial hibernation," vol. 34, no. 27, Jul 2013, pp. 2020–2021.

5. Pibarot, P., & Dumesnil, J.G., "The Relevance of Prosthesis-Patient Mismatch after Aortic Valve Replacement". Nat Clin Pract Cardiovasc Med. 2008;5(12):764–765.

6. Rahimtoola, S.H., "The Problem of Valve Prosthesis-Patient Mismatch," Circulation. 1978;58:20–24, Jul 1978.

7. "The 50 Best Mayo Clinic Doctors. Ever." – Hospitals, SYN, MedCity News, https://medcitynews.com/2011/12/the-50-best-mayo-clinic-doctors-ever

8. Holley, Joe. "Ayub K. Ommaya, 78; Neurosurgeon and Authority on Brain Injuries". Washington Post. 14 July 2008, www.washingtonpost.com/wp-dyn/content/article/2008/07/13/AR2008071301791.html

9. Rimal Hanif Dossani, Piyush Kalakoti, Jai Deep Thakur, Anil Nanda, Ayub Khan Ommaya (1930-2008): Legacy and Contributions to Neurosurgery, Neurosurgery, Volume 80, Issue 2, February 2017, Pages 324–330, https://doi.org/10.1093/neuros/nyw031

10. Watts, G. "Ayub Khan Ommaya" Obituary, The Lancet, vol. 372, no. 9649, pp. 1540, Nov 2008, https://doi.org/10.1016/S0140-6736(08)61642-6

11. Dewan, M.C., et al. "Estimating the Global Incidence of Traumatic Brain Injury". J Neurosurg. 2018 Apr 1:1-18. https://doi.org/10.3171/2017.10.JNS17352.

12. "Advancing Peripheral Intervention Starts with me". https://startswithme.com/bolia/bolia.html

13. P.P. Goodney, A.W. Beck, J. Nagle, H.G. Welch, R.M. Zwolak. "National trends in lower extremity bypass surgery, endovascular interventions, and major amputations" J. Vasc. Surg., 50 (2009), pp. 54-60, https://doi.org/10.1016/j.jvs.2009.01.035

14. Selmon, M. "Peripheral Vascular Disease, Chronic Total Occlusion of the Peripheral Arteries". Center Disease Control. www.cdc.gov/nchs/data/icd/att3_cto_sep06.pdf

15. Kenge, AP, Echouffo-Tcheugui, JB. "Differential Burden of Peripheral Artery Disease". The Lancet: Global HealthI, vol. 7, no. 8, pp. 980-1, Aug 2019. https://doi.org/10.1016/S2214-109X(19)30293-1

16. "Aziz Sancar, Facts". The Nobel Prize. www.nobelprize.org/prizes/chemistry/2015/sancar/facts

17. Rogers, K. "Aziz Sancar: Turkish-American Biochemist". Encyclopedia Britannica, 4 September 2019. www.britannica.com/biography/Aziz-Sancar

18. Zagorski, N. "Profile of Aziz Sancar". PNAS, vol. 102, no. 45, pp. 16125-16127, Nov 2005. https://doi.org/10.1073/pnas.0507558102

19. Savarese, Gianluigi, and Lars H Lund. "Global Public Health Burden of Heart Failure." Cardiac failure review vol. 3,1 (2017): 7-11. doi:10.15420/cfr.2016:25:2

20. Kwestan. "From Goats to Artificial Hearts: The Story of Dr. Mussivand". Medya Magazine. https://medyamagazine.com/from-goats-to-artificial-hearts-the-story-of-dr-mussivand

21. Homa, A. "The Kurdish Inventor of Hearts". Rudaw, 1 October 2014, https://rudaw.net/english/world/10012014

22. "Prevalence". National Fibromyalgia Association. www.fmaware.org/about-fibromyalgia/prevalence/#:~:targetText=Fibromyalgia%20is%20one%20of%20the,children%20of%20all%20ethnic%20groups.

23. Fitzcharles, Mary-Ann, and Muhammad B Yunus. "The clinical concept of fibromyalgia as a changing paradigm in the past 20 years." Pain research and treatment vol. 2012 (2012): 184835. https://doi.org/10.1155/2012/184835

24. "Data & Statistics" – Venous Thromboembolism (Blood Clots), Centers for Disease Control and Prevention. www.cdc.gov/ncbddd/dvt/data.html

25. Hussain, A, "Kazi Mobin-Uddin, 1930-1999". Journal of Vascular Surgery, Volume 32, Issue 2, 406 – 407, Aug 2000.

26. McElrath, KJ. "Medical Use of IVC Filters Declines Worldwide – But is Still High in the U.S." Drug Safety News. 22 July 2017, https:/drugsafetynews.com/2017/07/22/medical-use-ivc-filters-declines-worldwide-still-high-u-s

27. "Edwards Lifesciences Enters into Agreement to Acquire CardiAQ" 10 July 2015. www.edwards.com/ns20150710

28. "Adel Mahmoud, global health leader and Princeton faculty member, dies at 76" The Office of Comunication, 13 June 2018, www.princeton.edu/news/2018/06/13/adel-mahmoud-global-health-leader-and-princeton-faculty-member-dies-76

29. "Human Papillomavirus (HPV)" World Health Organization, 11 April 2018. www.who.int/immunization/diseases/hpv/en/#:~:targetText=Human%20papillomavirus%20(HPV)%20causes%20cervical,12%25%20of%20all%20female%20cancers.

30. "Nature Index" Nature Index 2019 Biomedical Sciences | Supplements | Nature Index. www.natureindex.com/supplements/nature-index-2019-biomedical-sciences/tables/overall

31. Craine, AG. "Elias Zerhouni" Encyclopedia Britannica, 07 October 2019. www.britannica.com/biography/Elias-Zerhouni

32. "Episode 16: Elias A. Zerhouni, MD, Leading History." Radiology Leadership Institute, American College of Radiology, 9 Dec. 2019, www.acr.org/Practice-Management-Quality-Informatics/Radiology-Leadership-Institute/Resources/Leadership-Insider-Podcasts/Ep16-1912. "Elias A. Zerhouni, M.D." National Institutes of Health, 22 October 2015. www.nih.gov/about-nih/what-we-do/nih-almanac/elias-zerhouni-md

33. "Elias A. Zerhouni Biography" Encyclopedia of World Biography. www.notablebiographies.com/newsmakers2/2004-Q-Z/Zerhouni-Elias-A.html

34. "Syed Modasser Ali: Surgeon - Biography, Life, Family, Career, Facts, Information". PeoplePill. https://peoplepill.com/people/syed-modasser-ali

35. "20 Most Innovative Surgeons Alive Today". Healthcare Administration Degree Programs, 02 August 2019. www.healthcare-administration-degree.net/20-most-innovative-surgeons-alive-today

36. Rosch, J, et. al. "The Birth, Early Years, and Future of Interventional Radiology". Journal of Vascular and Interventional Radiology, vol. 14, no. 7, pp. 841-3, 2003. https://doi.org/10.1097/01.rvi.0000083840.97061.5b

37. "Coronary Stent Complications". Michigan Medicine: Cardiac Surgery. https://medicine.umich.edu/dept/cardiac-surgery/patient-information/adult-cardiac-surgery/adult-conditions-treatments/coronary-angioplasty-stenting

38. Mehlinger, S. "Visionaries, Alam Nisar Syed". Long Beach Business Journal. 02 December 2018. www.lbbusinessjournal.com/visionaries-alam-nisar-m-syed-health-care

39. "Worldwide Cancer Data", Worldwide Cancer Research Fund, 17 July 2019. www.wcrf.org/dietandcancer/cancer-trends/worldwide-cancer-data

40. "Radiation Therapy at MSK". Memorial Sloan Kettering Cancer Center. www.mskcc.org/cancer-care/diagnosis-treatment/cancer-treatments/radiation-therapy/what-brachytherapy

41. "Types of ACE Inhibitors for Heart Disease Treatment", WebMD, 05September 2018. www.webmd.com/heart-disease/guide/medicine-ace-inhibitors#1

42. "Salim Yusuf PhD", Canadian Medical Hall of Fame, 01 January 1970. www.cdnmedhall.org/inductees/salimyusuf

43. "Salim Yusuf: global leader in cardiovascular disease research", The Lancet, August 2015, vol. 389, no. 9984. https://doi.org/10.1016/s0140-6736(15)61492-1

44. "Teepu Siddique", Encyclopedia Britannica, 29 January 2016. www.britannica.com/biography/Teepu-Siddique

45. Kugelman, M. "Chicago Zindabad!", DAWN.com, 11 April 2013. www.dawn.com/news/801863

46. "Advanced Cardiac & Vascular Centers"., Advanced Cardiac & Vascular Centers, 08 January 2020. www.advancedcardiacandvascular.com/about/our-providers/jihad-a-mustapha

47. Hamilton, T.F. "Profile: Surgeon and innovator Dr. Jihad Mustapha is known as 'The Leg Saver'", mlive. 23 May 2011. www.mlive.com/living/grand-rapids/2011/05/profile_surgeon_and_innovator.html

48. Mustapha, J. A., Katzen, B. T., Neville, R. F., Lookstein, R. A., Zeller, T., Miller, L. E., & Jaff, M. R. (2018). Determinants of Long-Term Outcomes and Costs in the Management of Critical Limb Ischemia: A Population-Based Cohort Study. Journal of the American Heart Association, 7(16), e009724. https://doi.org/10.1161/JAHA.118.009724

49. Armstrong, D. G., Swerdlow, M. A., Armstrong, A. A., Conte, M. S., Padula, W. V., & Bus, S. A. (2020). Five year mortality and direct costs of care for people with diabetic foot complications are comparable to cancer. Journal of foot and ankle research, 13(1), 16. https://doi.org/10.1186/s13047-020-00383-2

50. "Succeeding in Specialty Independent Care", Cardiac Interventions Today. https://citoday.com/2019/04/succeeding-in-specialty-independent-care

51. "Access gynlaparoscopy.com. Leader in laparoscopic and minimally invasive surgery - Resad Paya Pasic", Accesify. www.gynlaparoscopy.com

52. "Jafar Golzarian, MD", Fairview. www.fairview.org/providers/g/o/l/z/a/golzarianjafar-900070015

53. "Husain Sattar, MD", UChicago Medicine. www.uchicagomedicine.org/find-a-physician/physician/husain-sattar

54. Averett, N. "Wildly popular Pathoma course creates an unlikely celebrity in medical education", UChicago Medicine, 25 January 2018. www.uchicagomedicine.org/forefront/patient-care-articles/2018/january/wildly-popular-pathoma-course-creates-an-unlikely-celebrity-in-medical-education

55. "Huda Y. Zoghbi, MD", Texas Children's Hospital. www.texaschildrens.org/find-a-doctor/huda-y-zoghbi-md

56. Francesco Tomasello. Madjid Samii: a visionary, creative man and a world neurosurgery leader. World Neurosurgery. 2013;80:473-474.

57. O'Rourke, M. F. (1992). Frederick Akbar Mahomed. Hypertension, 19(2), 212–217. https://doi.org/10.1161/01.hyp.19.2.212

58. "Madjid Samii", Internetional Neuroscience Institute, 10 September, 2018. www.ini-hannover.de/en/madjid-samii

59. "Madjid Samii, M.D., Ph.D. Curriculum Vitae", Samii's Essentials in Neurosurgery. https://link.springer.com/chapter/10.1007%2F978-3-540-49250-4_1

60. www.pharmaceutical-journal.com/your-rps/nadia-bukhari-appointed-as-fip-global-lead-for-gender-equity-and-diversity/20207175.article?firstPass=false

61. "Afshin Gangi", Interventional News, 09 June 2016. https://interventionalnews.com/afshin-gangi

62. "Afshin Gangi", eMedEvents. www.emedevents.com/speaker-profile/afshin-gangi

63. "Amber Panagos & Dr. Muhammad Asim Khan", Spondylitis Association of America, 17 September 2018. www.spondylitis.org/This-AS-Life-Live/amber-panagos-dr-muhammad-asim-khan

64. "Muhammad Asim Khan, MD, MACP, FRCP", PRIME® Faculty Biography, https://primeinc.org/faculty/biography/158/Muhammad_Asim_Khan,_MD,_MACP,_FRCP

65. "Azra Raza, MD", Herbert Irving Comprehensive Cancer Center. https://cancer.columbia.edu/azra-raza-md

66. Myelopysplastic Syndrome", Mayo Foundation for Medical Education and Research. 27 October 2017. www.mayoclinic.org/diseases-conditions/myelodysplastic-syndrome/symptoms-causes/syc-20366977

67. "Azra Raza, MD". www.managingmds.com/reference-mds/faq-library-mds/41-azra-raza

68. "Mahmoud A. Ghannoum, PhD, EMBA", Case Western Reserve University School of Medicine Department of Dermatology. http://casemed.case.edu/dept/dermatology/Faculty/MGhannoum

69. Dvorak, P. "A renowned scientist wants to thank the stranger who helped him stay in America" The Washington Post. 16 September 2019. www.washingtonpost.com/local/a-renowned-scientist-wants-to-thank-the-stranger-who-helped-him-stay-in-america/2019/09/16/6e5ae3b2-d8a0-11e9-bfb1-849887369476_story.html

70. "El Sayed", Profile – Georgia Tech Chemistry & Biochemistry. www.chemistry.gatech.edu/faculty/El-Sayed

71. "Mostafa A. El-Sayed", Zewail City of Science and Technology. www.zewailcity.edu.eg/main/content.php?lang=en&alias=mostafa_a_el-sayed

72. Stewart, E. "Mostafa El-Sayed's Nano Scale Fight Against Cancer", InChemistry, 17 August 17 2017. https://inchemistry.acs.org/content/inchemistry/en/acs-and-you/el-sayed.html

73. www.ncbi.nlm.nih.gov/pubmed/?term=Ikram%20H%5BAuthor%5D&cauthor=true&cauthor_uid=8977357

74. Broughton, C. & Hayward, M. "Christchurch heart doctor recognised in Queens Birthday Honours", Stuff, 05 June 2017. www.stuff.co.nz/the-press/news/93299019/christchurch-heart-doctor-recognised-in-queens-birthday-honours

75. Higgins, J. "Pioneering physician Masood Akhtar got hearts beating the right way", Milwaukee Journal Sentinel, 09 May 2019. www.jsonline.com/story/news/2019/05/09/masood-akhtar-electrophysiology-cardiac-arrhythmia-heart-medicine/1139530001

76. "Selected Works of Masood Akhtar, MD, FACC, FACP, FAHA, FHRS, MACP", Authora Health Care. https://works.bepress.com/masood-akhtar/

77. "Dr. Mehdi Shishehbor", Crain's Cleveland Business, 09 March 2018. www.crainscleveland.com/article/20180310/NEWS/180319999/dr-mehdi-shishehbor

78. "University Hospitals Appoints Mehdi H. Shishehbor, DO, PhD, MPH as New Director, Cardiovascular Interventional Center", University Hospitals Cleveland Medical Center, 11 July 2017. www.newswise.com/articles/university-hospitals-appoints-mehdi-h-shishehbor-do-phd-mph-as-new-director-cardiovascular-interventional-center

79. "Alexander Norbash, Professor and Chair, Radiology", UC San Diego Institute of Engineering in Medicine. https://iem.ucsd.edu/people/profiles/alexander_norbash.html

80. "Khalid Shah, MS, PhD", Harvard Stem Cell Instiute. https://hsci.harvard.edu/people/khalid-shah-phd

81. "Director", Center for Stem Cell Therapeutics and Imaging. http://csti.bwh.harvard.edu/director

82. "Miss. Rozina Ali M.D, FRCS (Plast), MB BS, BSc", Cadogan Clinic. www.cadoganclinic.com/miss-rozina-ali

83. www.rozinaali.com

84. "Ali Guermazi, MD, PhD PROFESSOR, RADIOLOGY", BU SCHOOL OF MEDICINE. www.bumc.bu.edu/busm/profile/ali-guermazi

85. "Ali Guermazi, MD, PhD President & Co-Founder", Boston Imaging Core Lab. www.bicl.org/ali-ii

86. "Expert: Arshed Quyyumi, Cardiology" Emory News Center. https://news.emory.edu/tags/expert/quyyumi_arshed/index.html

87. "Highlighted Researcher: Arshed Quyyumi", Emory Daily Pulse. www.emorydailypulse.com/2018/07/18/highlighted-researcher-arshed-quyyumi

88. "Arshed Quyyumi awarded for excellence in research", Emory Daily Pulse. www.emorydailypulse.com/2016/06/24/arshed-quyyumi-awarded-excellence-research

89. "Biography of Nawal M. Nour, MD, MPH", Brigham Health: Brigham & Women's Hospital. www.brighamandwomens.org/obgyn/african-womens-health-center/directors-bio

90. "Nawal Nour", The Commonwaelth Fund. www.commonwealthfund.org/person/nawal-nour

91. FTSC. "Famous Figures of the Modern Turkish Medical School", Muslim Heritage. 23 October 2007. https://muslimheritage.com/famous-figures-of-the-modern-turkish-medical-school

92. Yong Tan, S. "Hulusi Behçet (1889–1948): Passion for dermatology", Singapore Medical Journal, vol. 57, no. 7, pp. 408-409. July 2016. https://doi.org/10.11622/smedj.2016123

93. Tanguin, Y. "A Curious Binder for Blood Cells: Dr Hasan Reşat Sültdım (1884-1971)",Kanbilim.com, 01 July 2013. http://kanbilim.com/?p=2324

94. Mercer, S.T. "THE DERMATOSIS OF MONOCYTIC LEUKEMIA", Arch Derm Syphilol, vol. 31, no. 5, pp. 615-635. May 1935. https://doi.org/10.1001/archderm.1935.01460230002001

95. https://muslimheritage.com/uploads/poster_2.pdf

96. Barlas U. "Ord. Prof. Dr. Akil Muhtar Ozden (1877-1949): his life and his scientific contributions", Tip Tanhi Arastirmmalari, vol. 10, pp. 207-220. 2001.

97. Naderi, S., et. al. "Dr. Ahmet Münir Sarpyener: pioneer in definition of congenital spinal stenosis", Spine Phila Pa, vol. 32, no. 5, pp. 606-608. 01 March 2007.

98. "Combining Technical Skill with a Uniquely Designed Device for CTO Success" Cath Lab Digest, vol. 24, no. 12, December 2016.

99. "Mahmood Razavi MD, MS, FSIR, FSVM", Adventus Ventures. https://adventusvc.com/partners-advisors/mahmood-k-razavi-md-ms-fsir-fsvm

100. 1"Syra Madad, DHSc, MS, MCP." LinkedIn, LinkedIn, www.linkedin.com/in/syra-madad-dhsc-ms-mcp-5b9495.

101. 1"Dr. Syra Madad." 1A, WAMU 88.5 - American University Radio, 27 Jan. 2020, the1a.org/guests/dr-syra-madad.

102. 1"Pandemic: How to Prevent an Outbreak." (2020). [film] Directed by I. Castro, D. Mynard, R. McGarry and D. Shultz. Netflix.

El-Mofty: https://pubmed.ncbi.nlm.nih.gov/10098699

www.sciencedirect.com/topics/medicine-and-dentistry/psoralen

SH Weshahy:

Weshahy AH. Intralesional cryosurgery: A new technique using cryoneedles. J Dermatol Surg Oncol. 1993;19:123–126.

https://docksci.com/intralesional-cryotherapy-for-treatment-of-keloid-scars-a-prospective-study_5a69070c-d64ab20445382277.html

https://emedicine.medscape.com/article/1294801-overview#a4

https://pubmed.ncbi.nlm.nih.gov/26749491

Ghaus Malik: https://pubmed.ncbi.nlm.nih.gov/33045451

https://wedns.org/category/dandy-medal-recipients

Mark Humayan: https://keck.usc.edu/faculty-search/mark-s-humayun

https://theophthalmologist.com/power-list/2018/mark-humayun

www.nvisioncenters.com/education/eye-disease-statistics

https://hscnews.usc.edu/mark-humayun-elected-a-2016-fellow-of-the-national-academy-of-inventors#:~:text=Mark%20S.,accorded%20solely%20to%20academic%20inventors.

Mohiuddin: www.trtworld.com/magazine/a-pakistan-born-us-doctor-tries-to-save-human-lives-with-pig-hearts-51501; www.medschool.umaryland.edu/profiles/Mohiuddin-Muhammad

Azra Raza www.thethirdwayofevolution.com/people/view/azra-raza

Mahmood Hai hwww.simichigan.com/dr-mahmood-hai; www.muslimsforamericanprogress.org/an-impact-report-of-muslim-contributions-to-michigan

Adah Al-Mutairi: https://eluxnanolipo.com/about/management-team-leadership;

www.forbes.com/sites/michaeltnietzel/2021/07/03/meet-the-worlds-most-influential-women-engineers/?sh=5aa3ab5d34c0; https://web.archive.org/web/20170115223959/http://pharmacy.ucsd.edu/faculty/bios/almutairi.shtml

www.thenationalnews.com/mena/arab-showcase/2022/08/11/woman-of-substance-the-materials-world-of-adah-almutairi

Salimuzzaman Siddisui:

www.dawn.com/news/1050186

www.dawn.com/news/620754

https://royalsocietypublishing.org/doi/10.1098/rsbm.1996.0025

https://tribune.com.pk/story/695330/dr-salimuzzaman-siddiqui-the-man-who-merged-eastern-and-western-medicine/

Naweed Syed:

www.cprdc.ca/portfolio-items/syed-naweed/

https://pakobserver.net/dr-naweed-syed-a-pakistani-behind-invention-of-worlds-first-brain-chip/

Hayat Sindi:

www.abouther.com/node/2061/people/leading-ladies/hayat-sindi-trailblazing-sciences

https://education.nationalgeographic.org/resource/explorer-profile-hayat-sindi-biotechnologist/

Mohammed Mohiuddin:

www.betterhealthcaretechnology.org/implementing-spatially-fractionated-radiation-therapy-sfrt-techniques-for-palliative-treatment-of-bulky-tumours/

www.cambridge.org/core/journals/expert-reviews-in-molecular-medicine/article/abs/divide-and-conquer-spatially-fractionated-radiation-therapy/E238317F5580299C51FBF749E7EDE9E2

Chang, Sha. A journey to understand SFRT (invited article for medical physics journal 50th anniversary special issue 2023) Feb 1, 2023.

www.youtube.com/watch?v=7BBykpO65ac